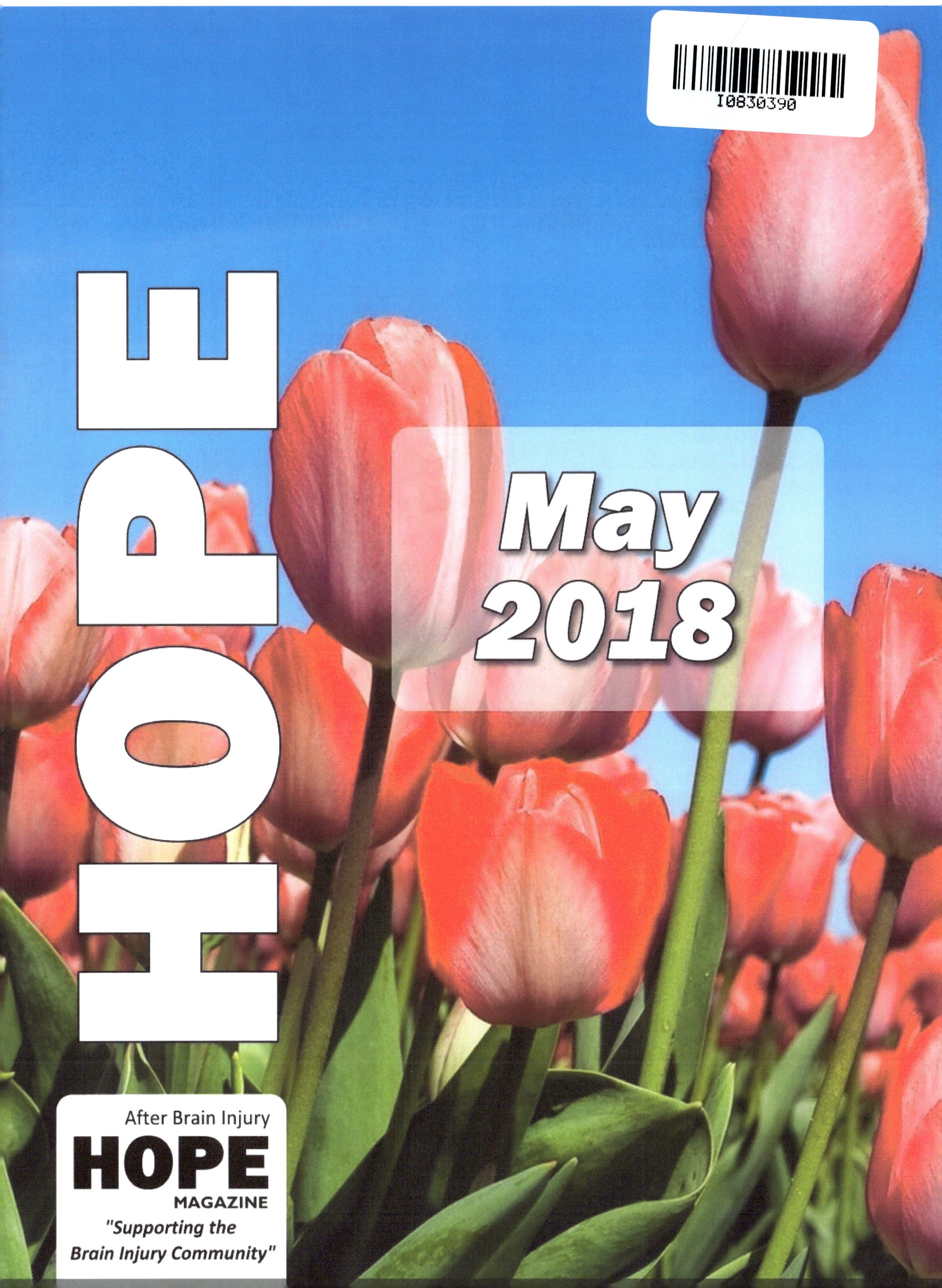
I0830390
HOPE
May 2018
After Brain Injury
HOPE
MAGAZINE
"Supporting the
Brain Injury Community"

Welcome

HOPE MAGAZINE

Serving All Impacted by Brain Injury

May 2018

Publisher
David A. Grant

Editor
Sarah Grant

Cartoonist
Patrick Brigham

Contributing Writers
Janet Baker
Nicole Bingaman
Aimee Champion
Deb Crowe
Darron Eastwell
Ted Stachulski
Taube Lubart Vallabha
Lisa Yee

*FREE subscriptions at
www.HopeAfterBrainInjury.com*

Welcome to the May 2018 issue of HOPE Magazine!

Over the last few weeks, I have had the opportunity to share with a couple of people that are new to the brain injury community. One was a fellow cyclist who, like me, was struck by a motor vehicle while cycling. The other is a childhood friend that I have known for over forty years.

Whenever I am in the company of someone new to this journey, I have to hold back a bit. There is so much I want to share, so many insights, strategies, skills, and more. These are life-saving tools I have found and used over the last seven years.

However, as brain injury survivors, it is far too easy to get overwhelmed with information overload. I know this from firsthand experience.

So I do as I've done for years, I keep it simple and I share three words that I clung to early on.

"It gets better."

Everyone has their own unique "better," but for most of us, time is a friend.

I hope you find something in this month's issue that helps you on your journey.

Peace,

David A. Grant
Publisher

Contents

What's Inside

May 2018

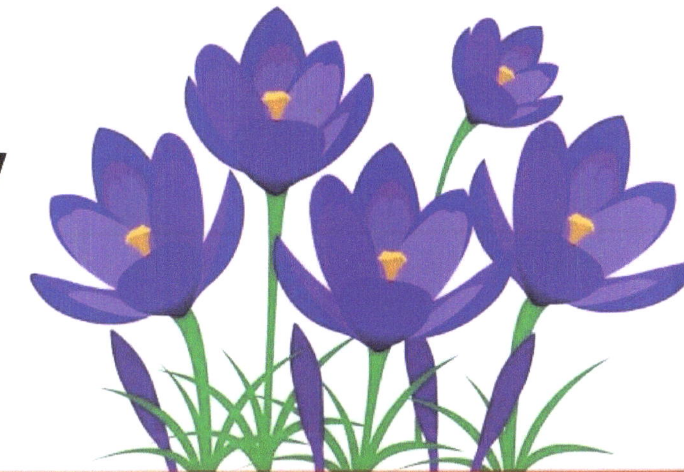

"Be happy for this moment. This moment is your life."

~Omar Khayyam

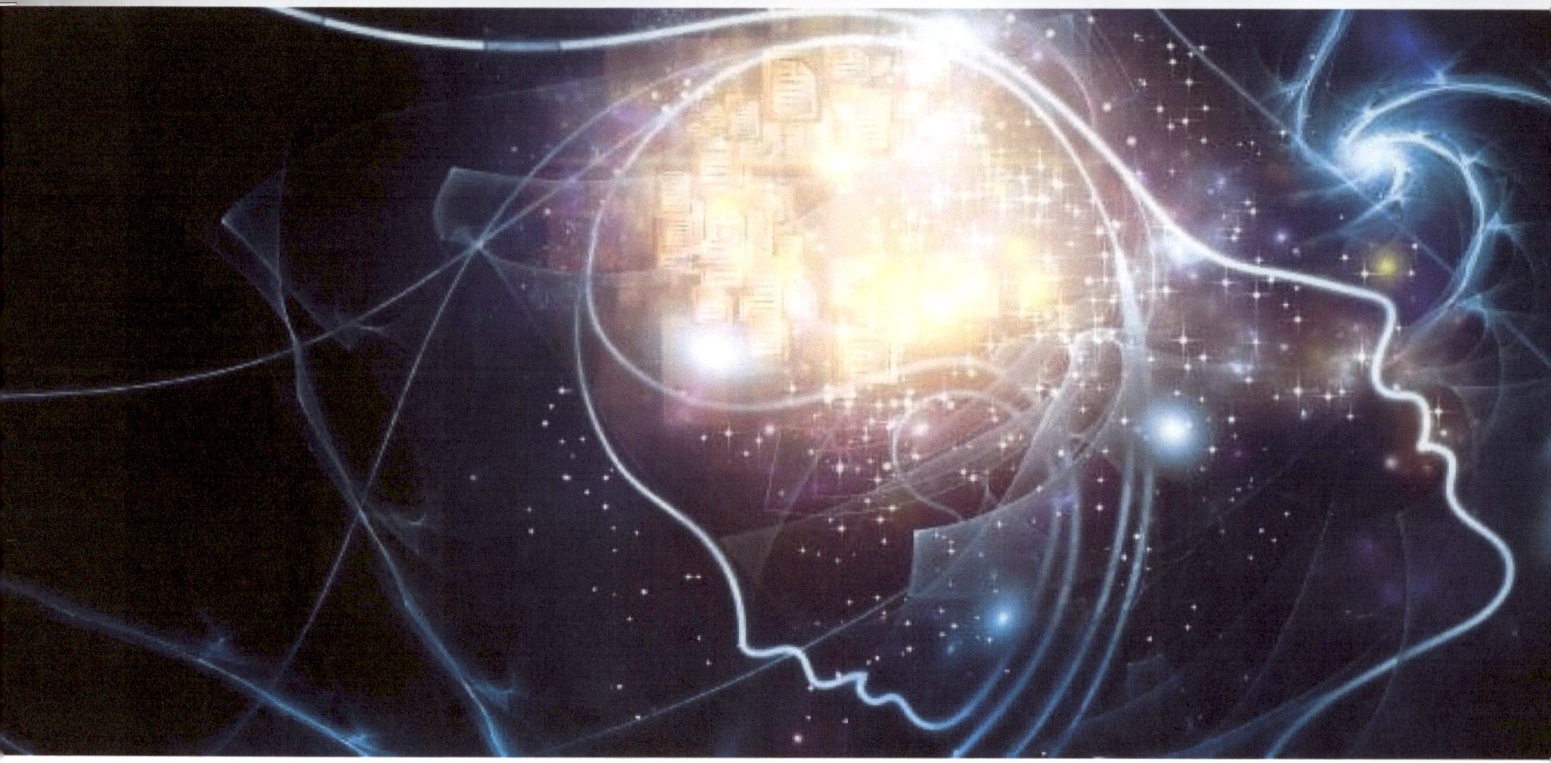

A Mother's Intuition
By Deb Crowe

It was a beautifully sunny Sunday afternoon in 2013. I had just returned from a baby shower to meet with my family after their lovely day of boating on Lake Erie. My daughter, Christine, was eager to get home and finish an essay due at school. She was rushing to pack the car and ensure she had all of her belongings as her mind was fixated to get home and meet her senior year academic deadlines.

Mothers have intuition. I believe it. I feel it. Before she left, I asked her to slow down. I reminded her that she had only a one-hour drive to get back home, with more than enough time to finish her essay and submit it online to her teacher.

As her car pulled away, I felt an intuition in the pit of my stomach. I looked up at the sky and sent a prayer to my father who passed away in 1987. I asked him, please, to watch over his granddaughter as she drove home.

> "Mothers have intuition. I believe it. I feel it. Before she left, I asked her to slow down."

Twenty-five minutes later my husband's cell phone rang. It was the Ontario Provincial Police. An officer gave us the news that our daughter had been in a car accident and was being transported by ambulance to the nearest hospital in Ingersoll, Ontario. My earlier hint of anxiety was now full-fledged, palpable fear, coursing through my body and spirit.

We learned that Christine had rolled her car into a ditch. My heart sank down to the bottom of my stomach. Our friends offered to pack up our boat and advised us to go. I was in shock. Was I Mom or case manager? This time it was not a client I would be helping, but my beloved daughter.

On the way to the hospital, we stopped at the accident scene to retrieve Christine's belongings from the car. I was in shock. My case manager's brain was pondering the logistics and the potential extent of Christine's injuries. But my brain as a mother was focused intently on keeping myself together so that I could be useful. My adrenaline-infused mind raced back and forth between logic and emotion, as I pondered what I would see at the Emergency Department.

When we arrived, the police officer was there and Christine – wearing a neck brace - was on a stretcher. She was pure white, like a blank piece of paper, with cuts on her arms and hands from the broken windshield. Again, my mind shifted from being an objective case manager, fully knowing the steps that lay ahead for Christine, while also being a loving mother trying her best to be calm and keep it all together.

Christine was diagnosed with a severe concussion and sent home. Her CT scan was normal. But, she did not look good, nor was she acting like herself, complaining of neck pain as we hastened to take her safely back home.

The next morning: definite pain in her neck and a droopy left eye. Even more frightening, when she started to speak, the left side of her mouth showed a definite droop.

My adrenaline-infused mind raced back and forth between logic and emotion, as I pondered what I would see at the Emergency Department.

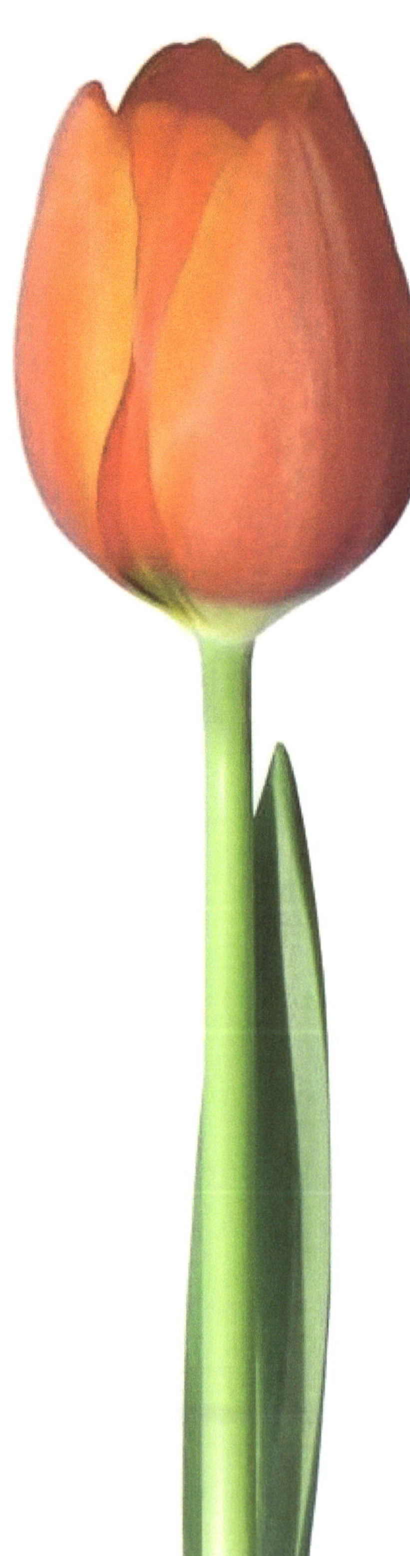

Enter case manager brain, and off to Children's Hospital Emergency we go, for a fast MRI just ten minutes after we arrived. The pediatric neurologist was very concerned. She diagnosed Christine with a mild traumatic brain injury but was also concerned with my daughter's slurred speech, the look of her eyes, her sensitivity to light, neck pain, plus the 'typical' symptoms that come with mild traumatic brain injury.

The next stage was our teenager, struggling not to believe that anything had happened and hoping to ward off any need for medical rehabilitation. Seeing your daughter's personality change is heart-wrenching. The "F"-word was now a part of Christine's everyday conversations.

Anger, frustration, depression and all the emotional 'feels' that come with brain injury were present. It's a much different scenario when it's your child and not a claim number attached to a lawyer and insurance company. Your daughter is your every single moment; a 24/7. You live your day moment by moment. Christine finally hit rock bottom and was ready to engage in medical rehabilitation in 2015, after her first attempt at post-secondary education. She attempted to try college and lasted a mere four weeks. Nothing was easy.

Now I understand first-hand what my clients and their families have gone through, along with the emotional and financial distress it caused them. There's no such thing as a non-biased medical assessment. One loses trust in the world and medical practice, in an industry that's become jaded as various so-called "professionals" seek to manipulate the system. The result these days is a long, drawn-out process, with a sorry lack of trust by the very people who most need therapy and support within their first two years of recovery.

Working in the healthcare industry since 1990, I have seen a lot, learned a lot, and ridden the unsteady waves of provincial legislation. If you have had, as I have, the best education that the province can offer and the privilege of helping so many families, your general state of mind is to feel well-versed and confident in your knowledge. But not when it's your child, and you're on the front lines, vying for every possible help.

Fighting the good fight is exhausting and defeating. Before 2010, we had terrific automobile insurance policies. After the legislative changes that year, the plans changed to a "base" menu with "extras" to purchase in an attempt to restore the original automobile insurance policy terms once offered. Having purchased all the "extras" does not necessarily mean, when you have a claim, that you actually can use them or be reimbursed. If you do the homework for you and your family, I'll bet you'll uncover the same disappointing result.

Having a claim is no guarantee: the people you expect to turn to for support for you and your family simply may not be there for you! Many families can relate to this. The insurance world is vast and connected. If you're on the receiving end of negotiating with an insurance company, don't be surprised if you experience some disappointment.

Fast forward five years to 2018. Christine has permanent symptoms that require attention from professionals who know, understand, and are well-educated in vestibular rehabilitation. She wears hearing aids and prisms in her eyeglasses, fighting physical, cognitive and visual fatigue every day.

The good news is that she is still here. She is a fighter. Her ongoing mantra is now about tenacity: to continue to grow, get better, and be the best that she can be each day. Her previous dream of being a trauma nurse may no longer be realistic.

> **We have worked as a family to love and support Christine along the way with cheering every little milestone of progress.**

However, with confident thinking, a positive mindset, and dreams to help others in another capacity, she will continue to work towards her new dream.

We have worked as a family to love and support Christine along the way with cheering every little milestone of progress. She has completed one year of college. Achieving that was hard and at times super challenging, but one has to push to succeed.

She has been accepted into University, and her goals and dreams are still to work within a health-related field. We, as a family, know that she will succeed. When the medical rehabilitation team goes away, along with the physicians, specialists, lawyers, and insurance professionals, our family is always there, ready to help pick up the pieces and continue.

That is what most professionals do not see or realize - what really happens behind the scenes. I will be an even better case manager now, because I have lived on both sides.

From 1990 to 2013, I worked in vocational rehabilitation, return-to-work, and case management. However, I have honestly learned more in the last five years, from 2013 to 2018, using my case management skills to help my daughter, than I had from my twenty-three years as a professional, helping other families.

My message to professionals and families reading this is to pause and reflect. Brain injury is quite serious. It comes with many symptoms, some that show up early and others that present as time moves along. Remain vigilant and aware of every treatment and the sequence in which they are introduced. The neck is often forgotten. If your loved one has sustained a whiplash-associated disorder (WAD I or II), actively find the right "experienced" professional to assist you. It will make vestibular rehabilitation a lot smoother while decreasing symptoms and improving your loved one's quality of life.

Meet Deb Crowe

Deb Crowe works as a Health Care Case Navigator helping families, legal counsel, and insurance companies work with challenging claims. She actively navigates the medical rehabilitation system to ensure that her clients receive the proper treatment, despite financial hardship. She also is a motivational speaker and published author.

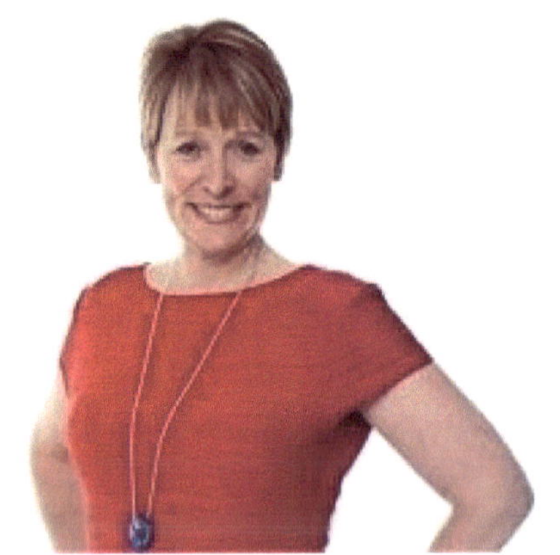

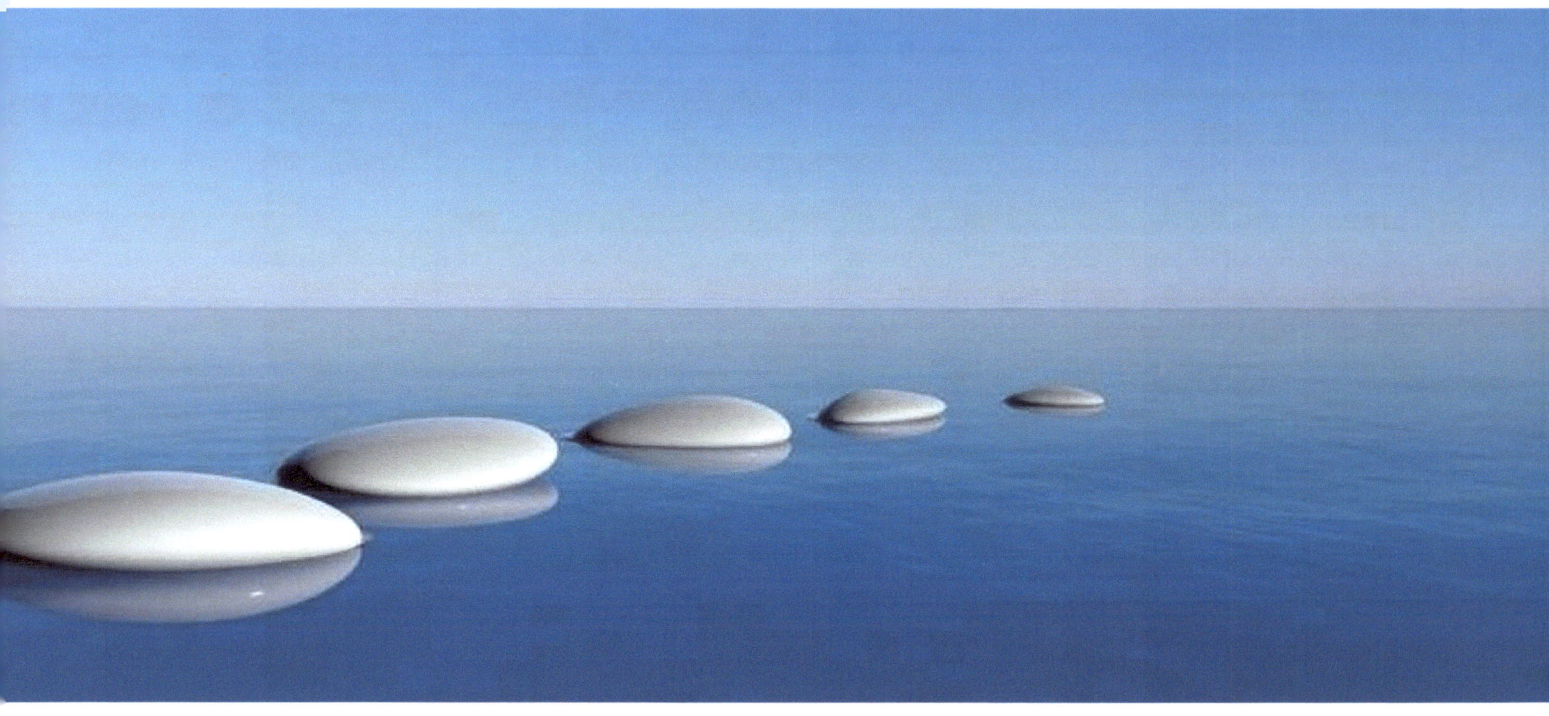

The Feeling of it All

By Nicole Bingaman

Driving to exercise class this morning I felt an unwelcome visitor come to my emotional door. This is something that we hear about survivors experiencing, but it happens to those who love survivors too. The term to describe this is "emotional flooding." This occurs when a surge of intense emotions arise that are difficult to ignore.

This morning the flooding came as I was driving to class, noticing the bend in the road. Suddenly I was assaulted by deep sorrow. I began weeping uncontrollably, feeling as if the worst of moments was upon me. My head filled with countless thoughts ranging from a sense of despair about how this happened to knowing that I could not change what did occur, and finally to wondering what our future might hold. These thoughts combined held a distinct impression of profound grief.

> "Something we must remember about grief is that it seeks to isolate us."

After parking, I attempted to pull myself together. I took a sip of cold water and drew some deep breaths. I pushed back at the feelings that were bothering me. Something we must remember about grief is that it seeks to isolate us. I have found that with ambiguous loss, the feelings of isolation can be more prominent because they are not as readily recognized.

Entering the studio, I looked like an absolute train wreck! Bloodshot eyes, wild hair, my nose running. Being true to myself, I didn't really care. It was 8:30 on a Saturday morning and I was proud to have shown up.

Friendly faces greeted me, and to my surprise, one of Taylor's dearest friends was there. Her presence was comforting, but I hoped she could not see my thoughts. I wanted to be okay, and I wanted the people around me to think that I was.

The first part of the class was dedicated to something called "pound," which involves cardio exercise using drumsticks and fun rhythms. It was perfect for releasing some of my pent-up tension. As I watched the instructor and tried to pick up the beat, I felt some of my despair diminish. It was a good time to get out of my own head.

I don't believe in suppressing emotions, but I also recognize that at times these feelings can be overrated. They can be released in a safe place before doing harm.

I floated in and out of the sequences, letting my mind and body escape. I welcomed the freedom of the distraction.

After forty minutes of pound, we transitioned to yoga. The first song that played rang true inside my head, "Wake me up when it's all over… when I'm wiser, and I'm older…" The flooding came again.

Were you ever in such a hard place that you wanted just to sleep through it? I've entertained the thought, "Wake me up when this is done; when all of the hard work, the efforts, and energy of healing is complete." It aligns with the part of caregiving that says, "This is too hard, I

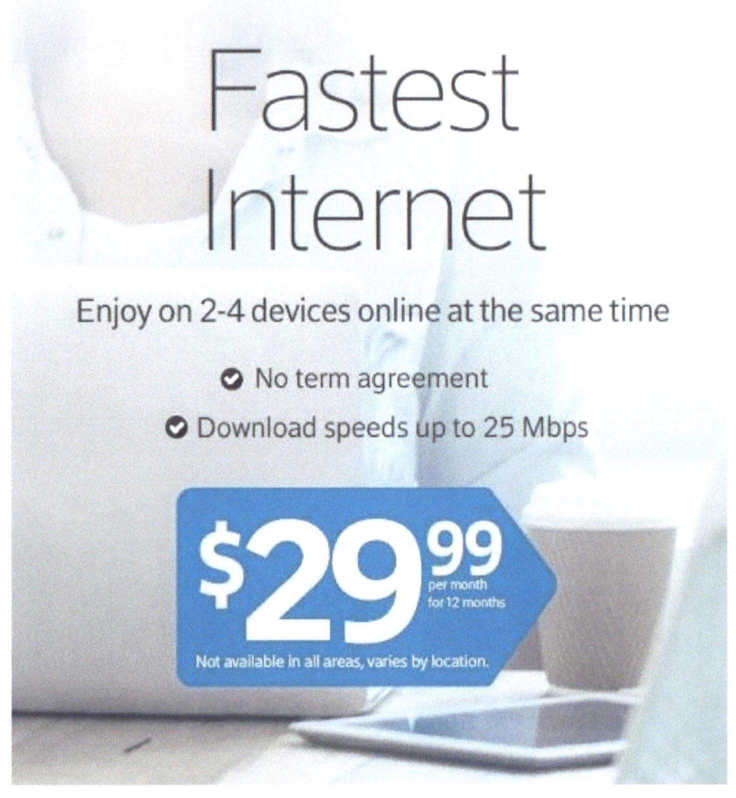

can't keep up." Someone once asked, "What is this?" In other words, "What do you feel like you can't do?"

This encompasses mountains and molehills. ***This*** defines things in caregiving that cannot be effectively explained, the ordinary and brutal moments making up our days. Sometimes ***this*** catches up with us, and we can't escape.

In listening to the lyrics of the song, I asked myself if I would really want to sleep through the hard days. Would I want to be in a position to not have to feel them? Would I choose an escape route if I could? And the answer is no. I wouldn't.

To feel is to be alive. To walk through the fire and to get to the other side is extraordinary. But you will get burned. Of course, we would choose not to have the fire if we could.

One of the things I ponder is the weeks that Taylor spent in a coma. His accident was on Thanksgiving Eve, and he first opened his eyes a month later. It was a while before he responded in any true sense to us.

Before Taylor's accident, he was in a strange place. He was twenty-one and figuring out life as an adult, relationships and the pressures of maturing.

Taylor had hit some pockets of normal struggling. One night, in particular, he was frustrated. He messaged me that he was having a difficult time, but wanted me to know he would be okay. He was going to figure it out.

Figuring it out felt good to him. Getting through hard moments is part of living.

During the weeks that he lay in the ICU void of any response, one of the things that resonated was that Taylor wasn't there in the same sense we were. I missed his presence within our family. I missed his hugs and his assurance to his father, his brothers, and I that things would work out. I want to be clear; I think it is normal to wish to escape the weight of responsibility that life with brain injury requires. It is normal to want for the challenges we confront to feel more comfortable.

This week I confided to a close friend, "Sometimes it hurts so much, I want to disappear." What I meant was this: I wish I could slip into a softer place, where the daily grind did not feel so demanding. A world of pink, fluffy cloudlike pillows, versus a bed of nails. In saying, "I want to disappear," I meant I want life to be easier. However, at the end of each day, I recognize that the whole of experiencing life is necessary. And this is a gift that some aren't offered.

When things get beyond hard, I challenge you to find a safe retreat. This can be in an exercise class, a song, contact with nature, or a good television show. But I also encourage you to find a place of gratitude. The feeling of it all is a gift, and aching is part of being alive. I truly don't think we would want it any other way.

Meet Nicole Bingaman

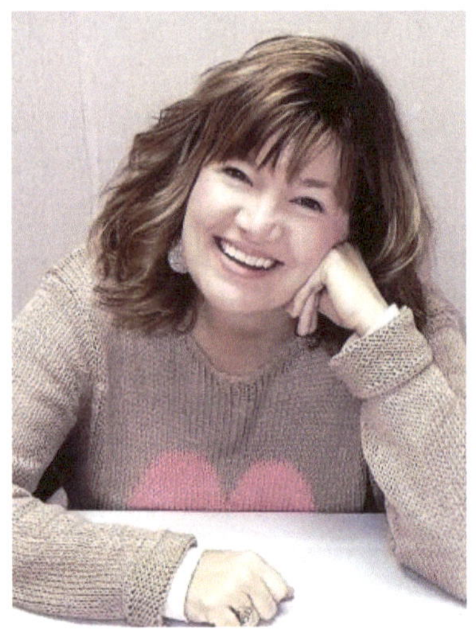

Nicole has worked in the human service field for over twenty years. Since Taylor's injury Nicole has become an advocate and spokesperson within the TBI community.

Nicole's book "Falling Away From You" was published and released in 2015. Nicole continues to share Taylor's journey on Facebook. Nicole firmly believes in the mantra that "Love Wins."

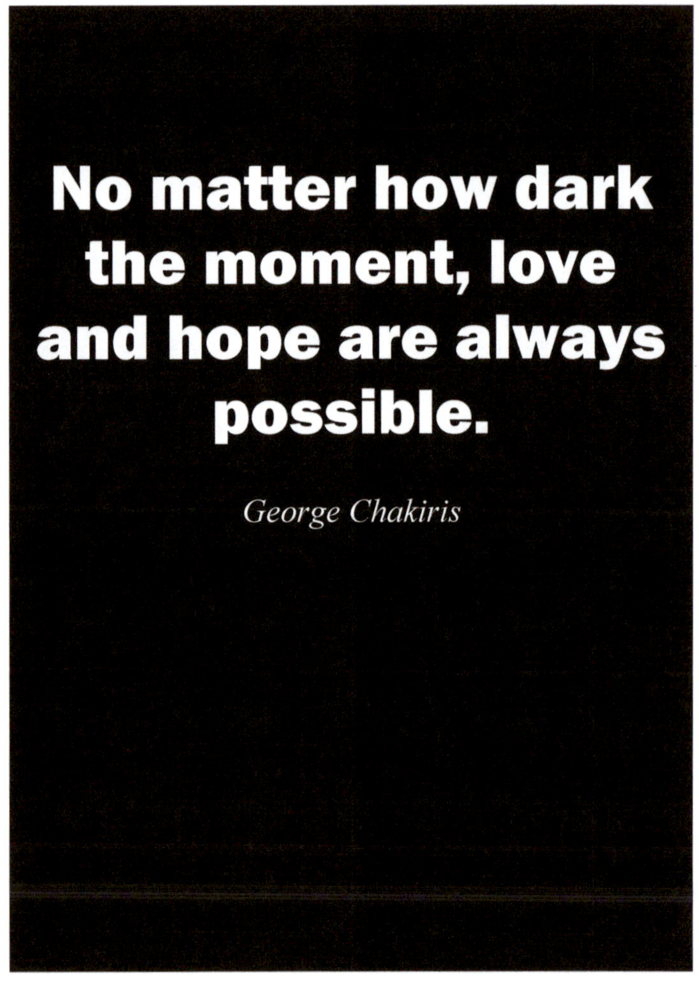

Gone

By Taube Lubart Vallabha, PhD

They say you don't know what you've got
Until what you've got goes away,
But when it comes to brain damage
What's gone tends to hide from what stays.
Your brain works by always comparing
Present input to memories from the past,
But if that past imprint gets damaged
And that part of you didn't hold fast,
Then what you're comparing things to now
Is something your brain invented
To compensate for the void created
When your brain became changed and lamented.
And now it's impossible to know
What parts of you used to be there:
The specifics of what is now missing
But still cries out to be shared.
But of course there's no way you can know this,
So you think what you know is what's real.
You rely on this false information:
It informs how you act and feel.
And so you become somebody
Quite different from who you once were,
Which might cause people around you
To wonder, "Hey, what's with her?"
But since you think you're still the same person
You might think that they're being rude,
And it's their fault you're having a struggle,
Or they're the one with the attitude.
It takes years for brain damage to heal.
If you're lucky that's what it will do.
And when that function returns
You'll have something to compare yourself to.
That's when you realize the loss
Of the person that you used to be,
The person you thought that you still were,
The one that you always called "me."
Then you can mourn what's been missing,
The knowledge of who you were then,
Because getting parts of yourself back
Means losing yourself all over again.

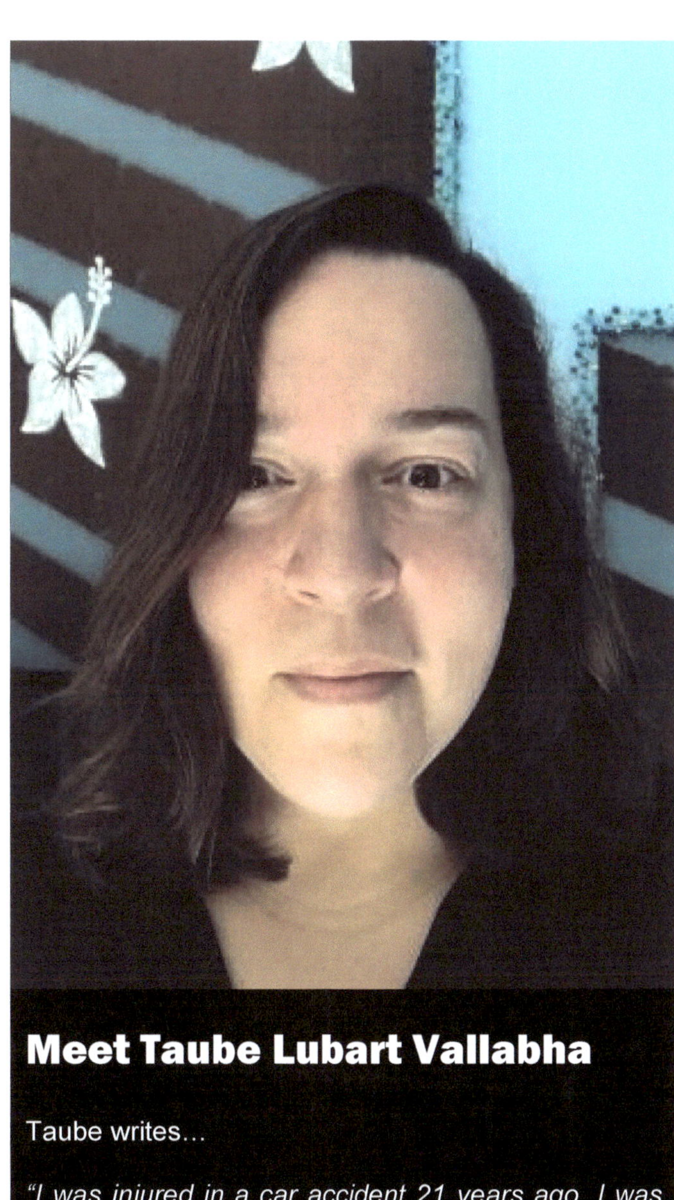

Meet Taube Lubart Vallabha

Taube writes…

"I was injured in a car accident 21 years ago. I was hyper-aware of the excruciating pain I was in, and it took me nearly two decades to figure out the extent of the brain damage I suffered. Ironically, at the time I was in grad school, studying Complex Systems and Brain Sciences.

I was somehow able to complete my PhD, and get married and have twins, too! Although I am still unable to work, I have regained most of the brain function I lost and have recently begun writing poetry inspired by my knowledge of the brain and brain damage on my blog at www.likeavortexinmycortex.wordpress.com."

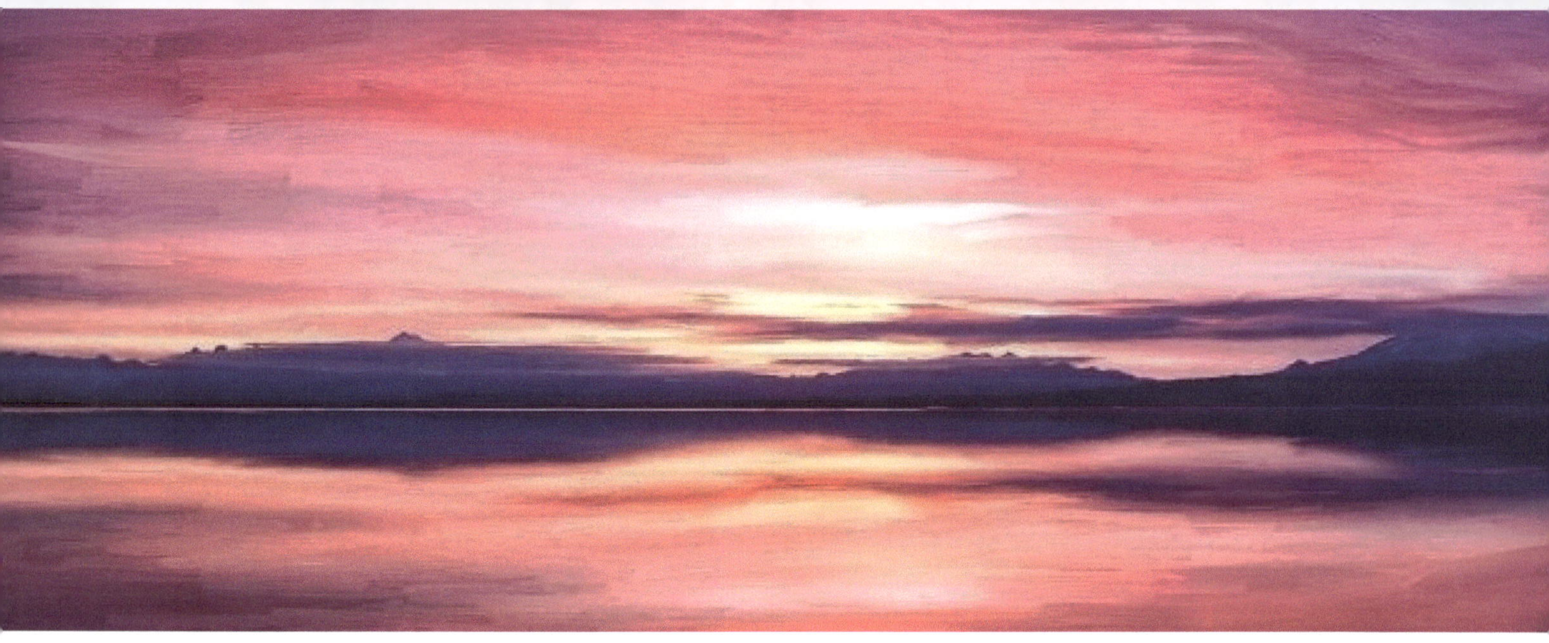

My Self-Worth Shift
By Aimee Champion

I recently needed to review my medical record from January 9, 2009, to present, with just over nine years of various documents. It has been an amazing journey - a traumatic one, but amazing, nonetheless. In those nine years, I watched from a cage within my body as my life slowly unraveled to reveal what I have always known. I am worthy.

It began with an arrogance of ego, wherein I relied upon science to bridge gaps in my DNA which were destined to cause breast or ovarian cancer - I had tested positive for the BRCA-II genetic mutation. I opted for a hysterectomy and an oophorectomy, together, commonly called, "total hysterectomy." Shortly after that, I opted for a double mastectomy with TUG Flap reconstruction. These were not uneducated or easily actuated choices. I did my homework, contemplated, discussed, and I gave my "informed consent."

> "Sometime between January 7 and January 9, in 2009, during the first of the breast arrest surgeries, I lost too much blood and died."

Sometime between January 7 and January 9, in 2009, during the first of the breast arrest surgeries, I lost too much blood and died. This was not acknowledged at the time. It would take six years for the knots of the threads that had defined my life to unravel, but they eventually would, releasing tremendous chaos.

During that time since "the incident," as each thread's tension gave way, a new (mis)diagnosis would be offered, new suspicions developed, and new accusations lodged against me. By this time, I was definitively the "problem." Eventually, in 2014 the reality of the circumstances had a name. I was diagnosed with an anoxic brain injury (fifteen randomly spaced white matter lesions) and small fiber peripheral neuropathy.

At the time, it was relieving, but that would not last long. To most people in my life, this diagnosis somehow demonstrated that by having a broken brain, I could not be deemed worthy again. I was damaged. There was no fix. But worse, I was incompetent and just needed to be spoon-fed "actual reality," unveiled from my "delusions."

Many attempted to help me by practicing tough love and telling it as they saw it. Here's how they saw it: "You are unworthy of my love," "You are unwelcome to participate with this family," "I cannot love you, I think you have borderline personality disorder."

As a result of these pervasive statements, attitudes, and behaviors toward me – as if I were garbage – I began to believe them. This drove me to a quite rational state of suicidal ideation wherein I honestly and deeply believed that all of these people would be better off without having to deal with me – "the problem." I even rationalized that I was incapable of being a mother, a role I purposefully sought by adopting my daughter.

> "I honestly and deeply believed that all of these people would be better off without having to deal with me."

Here is where the whole ordeal gets real. Having died, I finally understood the basis of faith. I finally realized that my journey does not define my worth. Worth is spiritually sourced, not materialistically owned. Today, I enjoy a state of wellbeing. I no longer grieve the lost me, but I do grieve my lost naiveté. It is not for me to determine the journey of others, but it is for me to stand steadfast in who I know I am. I have learned to see in the dark, and because of this, no human-derived light-switch can haunt me. I have no fear. I have only love for this experience and its softening of the edges of my ego.

I'm cautious, far more reliant on my intuition, but less judgmental, more open and authentic. It makes people, especially those who deemed me unworthy when I was injured, very uncomfortable. I take that as my invitation to use my steadfast sense of self as a beacon in the shadows of others; as a teacher, as an advocate, and as a guide. I am grateful this is the extent of discomfort for these students. After all, it can get so much worse. Although not nearly at full-time capacity, I have reinstated my license to practice law and I run a small law practice. I am a confident and competent mother. I am a darn good friend, especially to those who feel "unworthy."

The shift in my self-worth was dramatic but so worthwhile. In December 2008, I was a devout atheist. In January of 2009, I returned to this life a devout Buddhist. I practice the ancient tradition of Reiki.

I have gone from nine different pharmaceuticals (mostly ill-prescribed) each day, to zero. I have pain, and I have neuro-fatigue, but I also understand that these things do not determine the quality of my life. I believe that we create the quality of our destiny with each breath we take. I am worthy of each breath.

Meet Aimee Champion

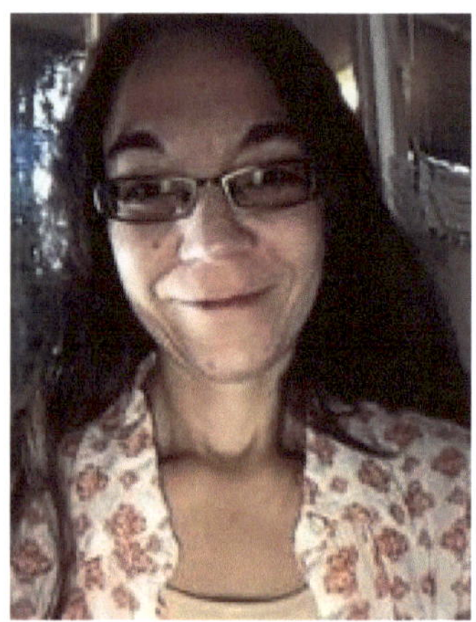

Aimee Champion is a woefully over-educated and experienced anoxic brain injury survivor. She operates a small solo law practice wherein her passion is empowering her clients to rebuild their lives after trauma. Aimee lives in Washington State with her co-parent, daughter and darling Daisy-dog.

Living With Hope

By Patrick Brigham

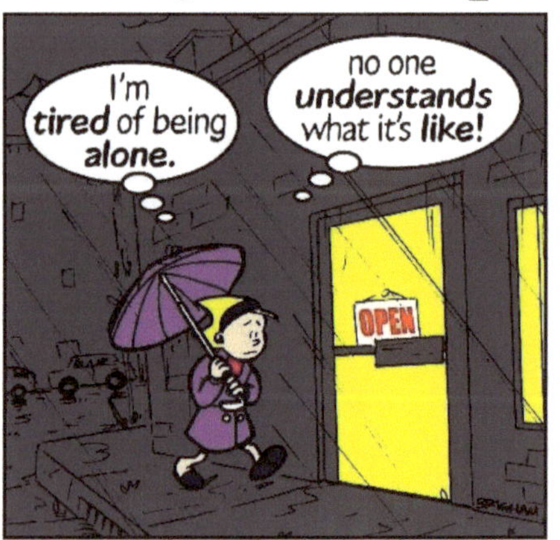

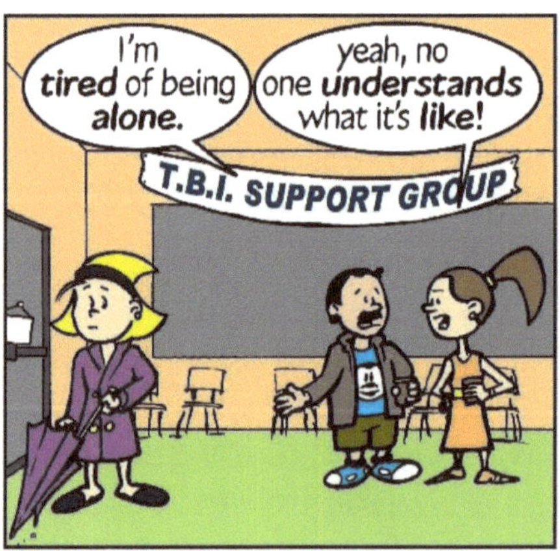

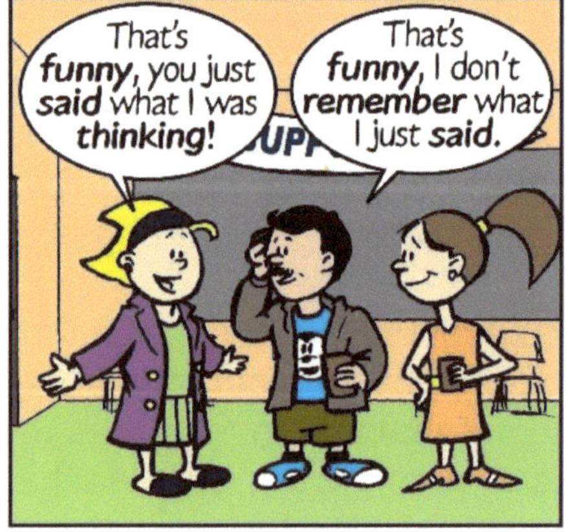

All My Ducks in a Row

By Lisa Yee

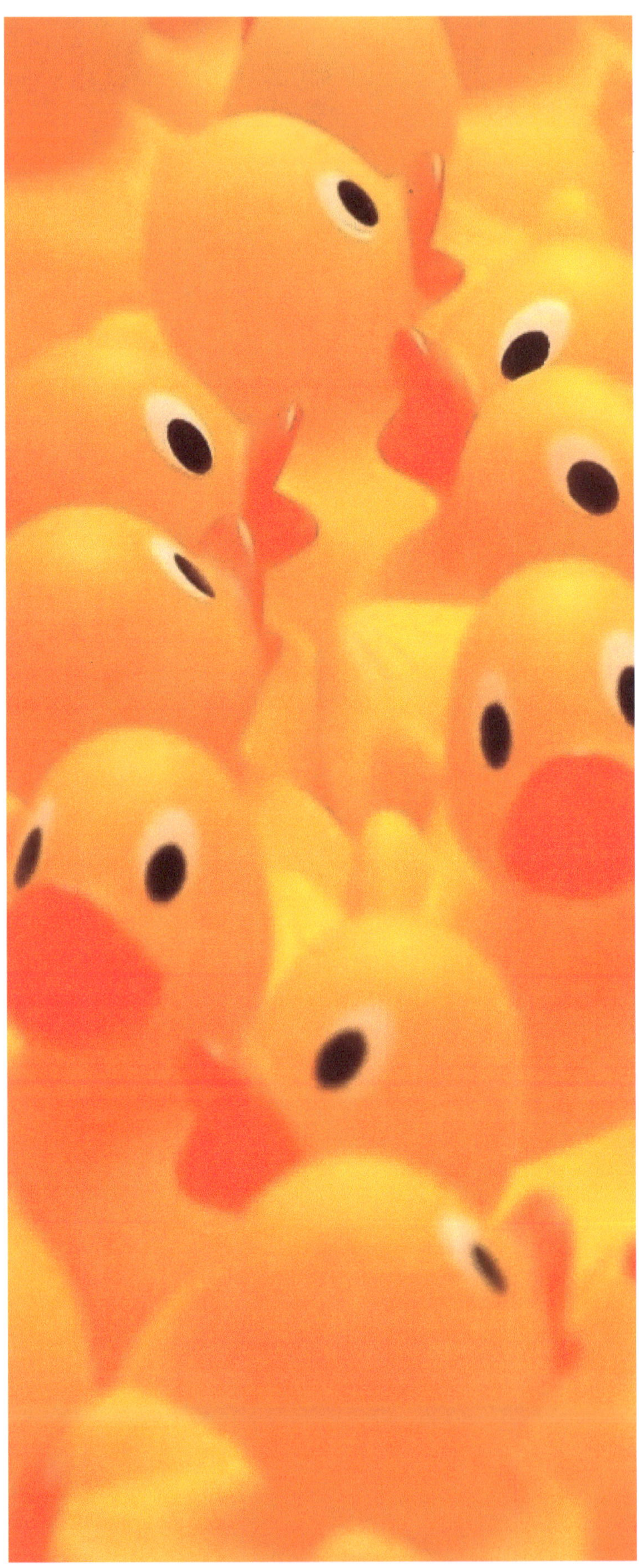

Our former neurologist once told my husband: "Lisa will be fine as long as all her ducks are in a row." In other words, things would be okay as long as nothing threw me off my routine.

As a TBI and epilepsy patient since a 2008 car crash, hoo-boy, did I have my routines! Sample day: Wake up, take my medication, eat breakfast, read the newspaper, exercise, shower and get dressed, eat lunch, nap, do minimal housework, have dinner, watch TV with husband, take my medication, go to sleep, take more medicine, and go back to sleep.

My life wasn't completely predictable; there was also the occasional seizure.

For the most part, my ducks remained in a row.

As the years went by, my life became fuller and happier, though still pretty regimented. I trained to become a yoga instructor and last year began volunteering as a teacher at a women's shelter and a veteran's center.

The article I wrote for my certification, "This Is My Brain on Yoga: From Injury to Enlightenment," was published in the March issue of TBI Hope and Inspiration, as well as in Meditation Magazine. I've always been the kind of person who tries to put on a happy face, even if I'm crying inside.

And my ducks and their rows?

Well, lately mine have been all over the place. Recently, I was stranded on the couch for two months while my foot healed from a fall down the basement stairs. (Life lesson: Do not carry a full basket of laundry down the stairs with both hands. Better still: Do less laundry.) My time on the couch led to a full-fledged mutiny on the duck row.

First, there was the situation at hand. For reasons too crazy to explain, when I lost my footing on the top step of the stairs, I had been wearing only a towel. Whimpering, I assessed the damage: toes curled under, bleeding knee.

I wisely decided to scoot to the freezer for a makeshift ice pack, then knocked the First-Aid kit off a shelf and patched myself up. Unwisely, I scooted to the dryer for something clean to wear, then scooted back.

Did I mention my husband wasn't home yet and my cell phone was upstairs?

Okay, I know it sounds like something out of "I Love Lucy," (of course, she'd have been wearing a robe), but back to my ducks.

Letting my broken metatarsal and ligament heal has meant canceling my volunteer yoga gigs and classes, and I'm having a hard time getting either place to reschedule. Plus, you wouldn't believe how the dirty laundry has been piling up. The thing is, I was finally able to walk, very slowly, to a yoga class today instead of getting a ride. And this is the first writing I've done in a month.

I still don't have my ducks in a row, but for now, I'm okay with my progress.

Meet Lisa Yee

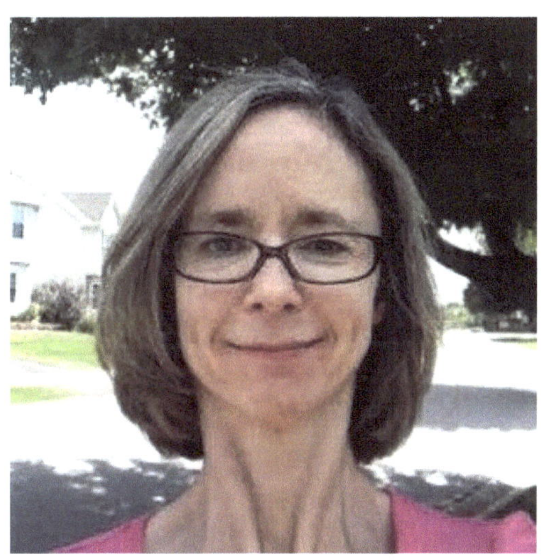

Lisa Yee of suburban Chicago suffered a traumatic brain injury/epilepsy in a 2008 car accident. Before her injury, she had been a newspaper editor for two decades after graduating from the Indiana University School of Journalism. It was there she met her husband, Ted. They have a daughter, Megan, of Chicago.

Post injury, Lisa became certified as a yoga instructor and now volunteers teaching yoga at a women's shelter and a veteran's center.

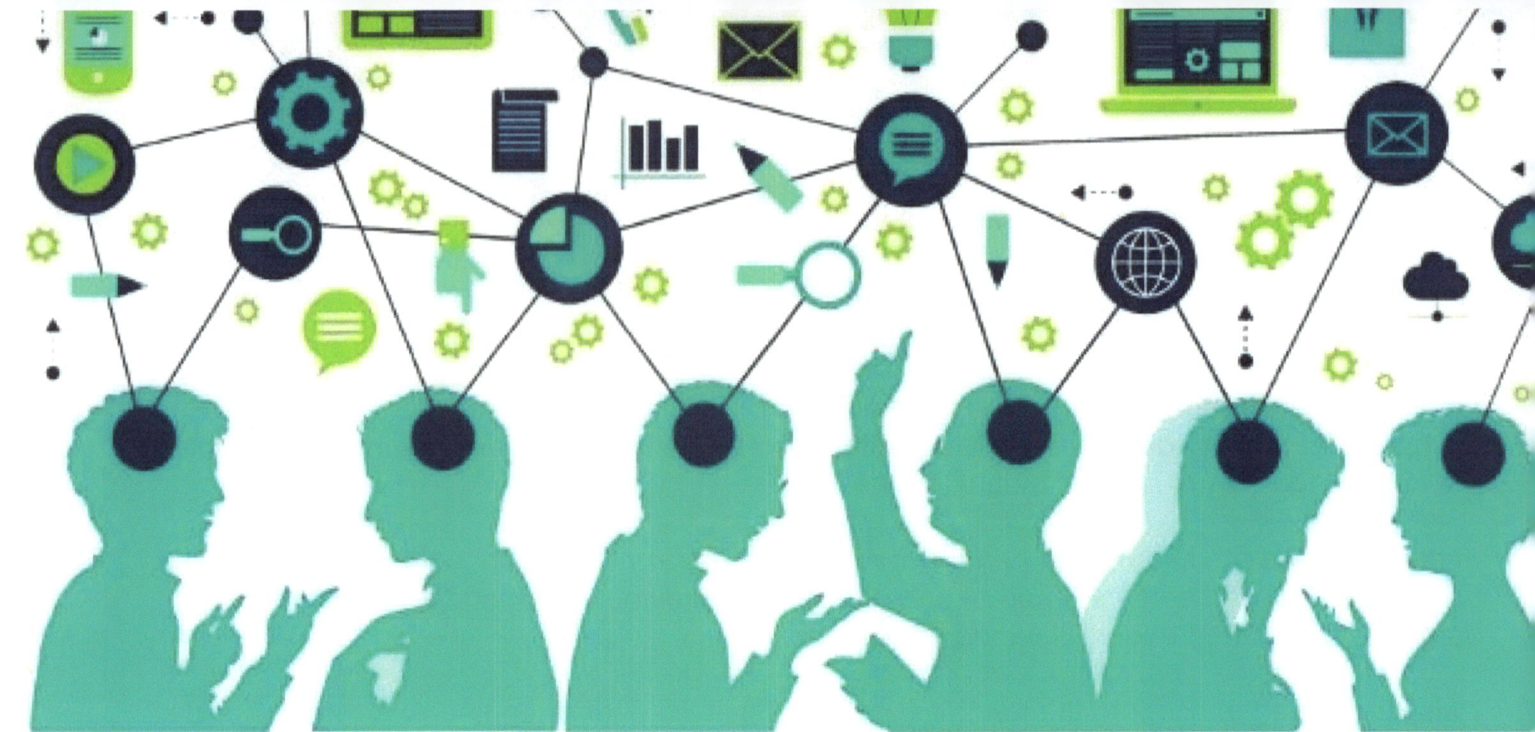

Learning to do Everything Again

By Janet Baker

My TBI occurred on October 21, 2011. That date is significant, of course, but there was a bit of history before that. My story begins sometime in 2009/2010. During those years, I went to the doctor several times with vague complaints. Nothing earth shattering, just weird. I always felt strange going in because I did not have any complaint to pinpoint. No significant pain or unusual symptom, just 'odd' stuff.

I had to 'think' about doing things that normally come naturally, like swallowing. I would cough/sneeze/hiccup more than normal. Over the course of two years, I went to physical therapy to work on a possible pinched nerve and had a colonoscopy to determine possible constipation issues.

> "I had to 'think' about doing things that normally come naturally, like swallowing."

Then I started getting severe headaches in the morning. Head-in-a vice kind of headaches! They would hit me as I was walking down the hall in the morning and would stop me in my tracks until they subsided. The only good thing is that they didn't last TOO long.

Most days when I would take my morning shower, I would be overcome with such a nauseating sensation that I would have to exit the shower and lay on the floor. Oddly enough, after being up for an hour or so and getting around, I would feel better and could go about my daily routine. However, it was obvious that what I was experiencing was far from routine.

While sharing my symptoms with my co-workers, one suggested that maybe I was pregnant. (In hindsight, that would have been a better diagnosis!) Finally, one morning as I lay on the couch waiting for 'normal' to find me, my husband asked if I was going to call the doctor or did he have to make the appointment for me. I once again went to the doctor. This time, he decided to send me for an MRI. With the addition of a headache symptom, he wanted to rule out an aneurysm.

On Tuesday, September 27, 2011, I went for an MRI. I had never been through one of those before so wasn't sure what to expect. When it was over, they told me to go to the waiting room. At this same time, my daughter, who had just turned 15, was with her dad and was getting her driving permit. She called me while I was in the waiting room and was very excited that she had passed. I told her how happy I was for her and that I would see her later that afternoon when she played volleyball. As I sat in the waiting room, the x-ray receptionist informed me that my doctor was on the phone. While standing there at the receptionist's desk, I was told that I had a brain tumor.

The time was about 4:30 PM. My doctor told me to come directly to his office and that he would be there until 5:00 PM. I drove across town in an absolute blur, not really understanding what was happening. When I got to the office, I was told that I had a tumor at the base of my brain and that it was serious.

"While standing there at the receptionist's desk, I was told that I had a brain tumor."

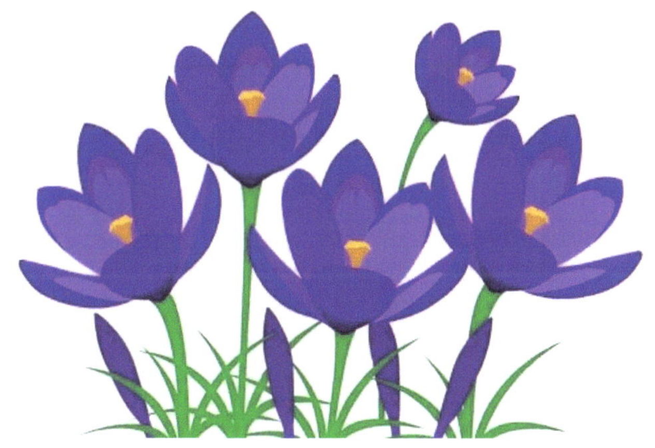

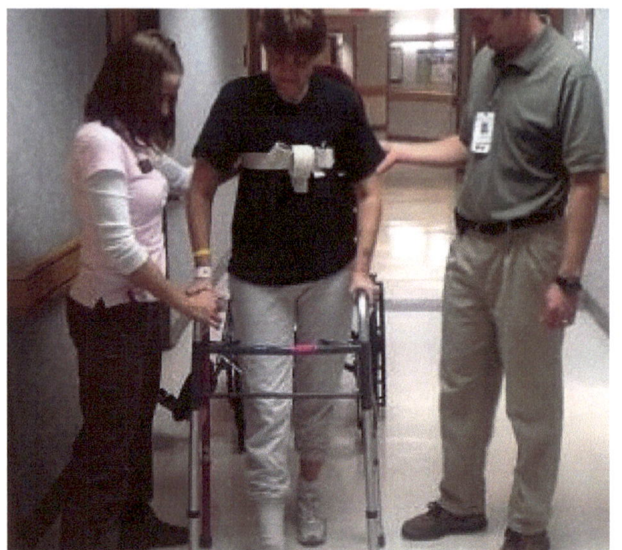

He recommended I see a neurologist as soon as possible. I left the doctor's office with a steroid prescription and drove to my daughter's volleyball game. While in the stands of a high school gym, I relayed my diagnosis to my husband. It was all so surreal.

On Friday, September 30th, I saw a neurologist. He told us the tumor was about 3 cm in size and was positioned at the base of my brain, at the top of my spinal cord (where there is not a lot of room). It is also the junction where MANY nerves intersect.

Surgery was scheduled for October 21st. Of course, as with all surgery, I was given the list of possible risks. In my case, some of those possibilities were potentially more likely and more devastating. There was a possibility that I could: be paralyzed, be on a ventilator, or die. There was also the possibility that the tumor could be cancerous which would naturally cause other issues. They would not know anything further until they performed the surgery.

The weeks leading up to October 21st were very much a blur. I spent the next three weeks telling parents, kids, family members, co-workers, and church members of my situation. I also posted my situation on Facebook. Through those connections, the infamous grapevine took care of relaying my story to anyone who might remotely want to know. I was 46-years-old. My kids were 15 and 20 at the time. My daughter was just starting her freshman year in high school. My son was in his second year at Technical school. My brother had just gotten married. I had a job that I loved at a local community bank.

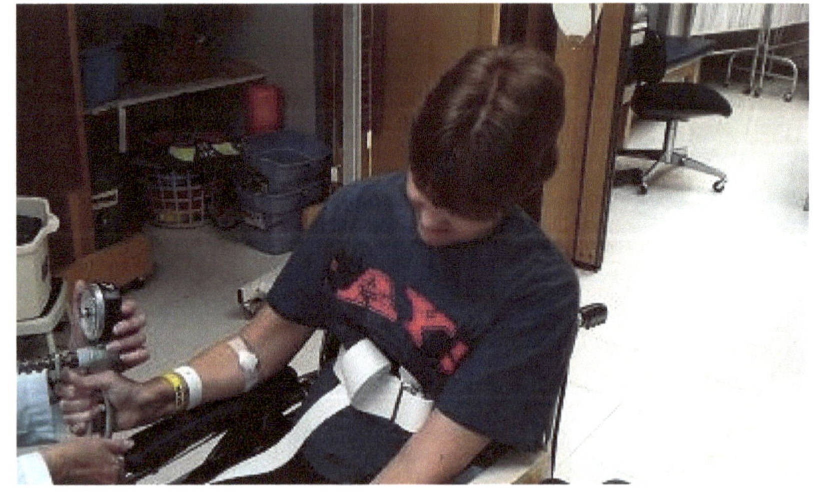

Having a brain meningioma was not in my plans in any way, shape or form. I spent a LOT of time talking, talking, and talking some more. I updated my coworkers on various projects I was involved in, along with what was still left to do. In my mind, I was planning to be out for six weeks and come back as my normal self (much as I had after having a baby). At home, I told my husband what bills needed to be paid and relinquished my Facebook password. (As a morbid side note, we did talk about other possibilities, including where I wanted to be buried.)

On the outside, I tried to live as much a 'normal' life as I possibly could. On the inside, my mind whirled with all kinds of 'what-ifs.'

Friday, October 21st, came much too fast. On October 20th, I went to my daughter's volleyball game (as usual). When we left, I hugged her and my parents and told them I would see them after surgery. I had to be at the hospital very early the next day. My daughter was going to spend the night with my parents, go to school as 'normal,' and then come to the hospital with my son when they got out of school.

We got to the hospital at the crack of dawn and prepared for a VERY long day. (Well, my husband prepared for a long day. I don't remember too much of it.) The surgery lasted for ten hours. Over the course of the day, all kinds of friends and family showed up (so I am told), to sit with Russ and support each other.

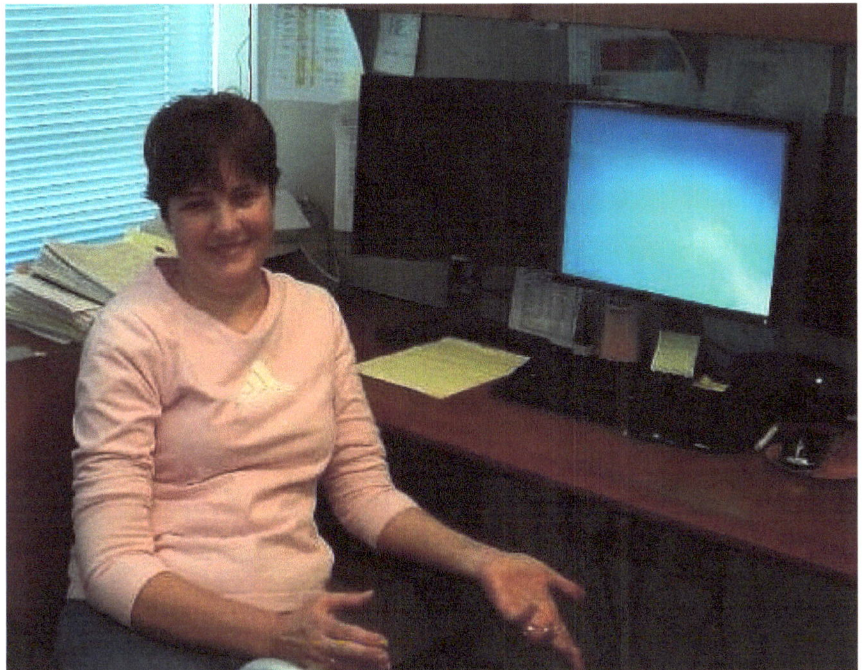

When I woke up Friday evening, I was in the ICU and had an upside-down 'J' stapled on the back of my head. I remember being curled into a fetal position and having a suction device taped to my hand (since I could not swallow). I think I barely woke up and they put me back to sleep. I remember only bits and pieces of the next few days. The highlights were that I could not swallow, hold my head up, or walk. I also had an extreme case of double vision. I spent three days in the ICU and another four days in the hospital. Since I was not able to swallow, I had a feeding tube surgically implanted. When I was released from the hospital, I was transferred to a rehabilitation center where I spent another thirty days.

I had to learn how to do everything again. I could not stand up. My speech was barely a whisper. My strength and dexterity were nonexistent. I needed help to do EVERYTHING. I couldn't go to the bathroom by myself and required assistance getting into a sit-down shower. I remember having difficulty even putting a 40-piece puzzle together. I did 'homework' in my room which consisted of first-grade penmanship sheets. Every ounce of my self-esteem was tested. I experienced severe arm bruising from the number of blood draws they did daily, and I ended up with pneumonia after vomiting and aspirating into my lungs.

I got to come home on a 'trial run' on Thanksgiving Day. I was still not able to swallow, so I spent that day in the recliner watching others eat. But being part of the holiday festivities allowed me to at least imagine something close to 'normal.'

I officially came home on November 29th. I still was not able to walk or eat. I continued out-patient therapy and tried to get some semblance of myself back. I graduated to a walker by Christmas and decked it in full holiday ornamentation, including lights! Four months after surgery, I went back to work on a part-time basis.

Today, it has been over six years since my diagnosis. I have several residual effects from either the tumor or surgery itself. Many are reminiscent of someone who has had a stroke. I have walking/balance issues. I used to go out after supper and walk several miles around the neighborhood. Now I walk like I am drunk. I worry about how far away something is or what the terrain is like to get there. I am unable to climb stairs without a rail or assistance and can't carry anything too significant. The nerve that innervates my right shoulder blade was damaged. My shoulder now juts forward, and I am limited how far I can lift my arm. I have lost temperature and pain sensation on my left side. My right vocal cord and part of my tongue are paralyzed. I am left with a soft voice and have a limited vocal pitch. My strength, dexterity, and neck movements are limited.

I still have 'pity parties,' where I grieve for the old me and miss the things that I am no longer able to do. I used to enjoy recreational sports such as bowling, tennis, skating, and ping-pong. I used to enjoy planting flowers in the beds around our house. Now I am able to get a few pots together. I don't walk in the yard at all unless someone is with me. However, with all the changes that have happened to me, I do think of the alternatives and realize how lucky I am. Comparing where I am now to who I was in the months after surgery is significant.

"I still have 'pity parties,' where I grieve for the old me and miss the things that I am no longer able to do."

My personality has changed. Some might say for the better, some might say for the worse. I know it is different; I can feel it. I cry more often at what may seem like silly things.

It changed my family as well. My kids grew up fast and had to deal with things I didn't remotely have to at their age. I am no longer the mom or the wife that I once was. We no longer pick up and go anywhere. There is always a concern of how I will be able to navigate new places. We are mindful of getting my disability hang tag if we happen to be traveling in a different vehicle. I still have trouble swallowing. I eat slowly, and I am always the last one done. I refrain from communion at church because I don't want to choke. And I don't dare try to swallow a pill. I am extra worried about things now. Every bump, bruise, pain, or anything unusual that I experience makes me wonder if I should worry.

I still work for the bank but in a much different capacity. I miss the old me and my old job. I used to thrive on the daily challenges and enjoyed what I did. I now have a job that allows me to use my skills differently and to work from home if the weather creates unsafe walking conditions.

Before my TBI I never actively thought about disabilities. Of course, I was aware that there were disabled people, but I was never around anyone to fully experience what that meant. While I thought I was sympathetic and empathetic before, now I see things through an entirely different set of eyes. I feel obligated to tell new people that I meet at least an abbreviated version of my story lest they think my physical limitations somehow transcend into limited mental capacity. (Maybe I am doing this to convince myself). I wonder what new people think when they meet me. I wonder if people I have known for years think about the 'old' me when they are with me now. There are many days that I still long for my prior life, however, I also realize that things could be even more different than they are now. I am thankful for all my friends and family who continue to support me and continue to work on being the best 'me' I can be!

Meet Janet Baker

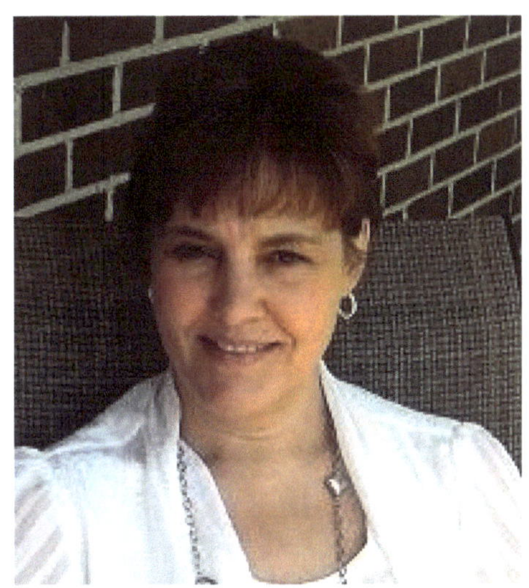

Janet Baker is a fifty-something wife and mother of 2 from Jefferson City, Missouri. Her TBI occurred in 2011 after she was diagnosed with and had surgery for a tumor at the junction of her brain and spinal cord. While she does still have a number of physical limitations, she leads a relatively normal life. She takes life at a much slower pace than she did previously and makes a lot of decisions based on her new mantra of 'life is too short-so don't sweat the small stuff'.

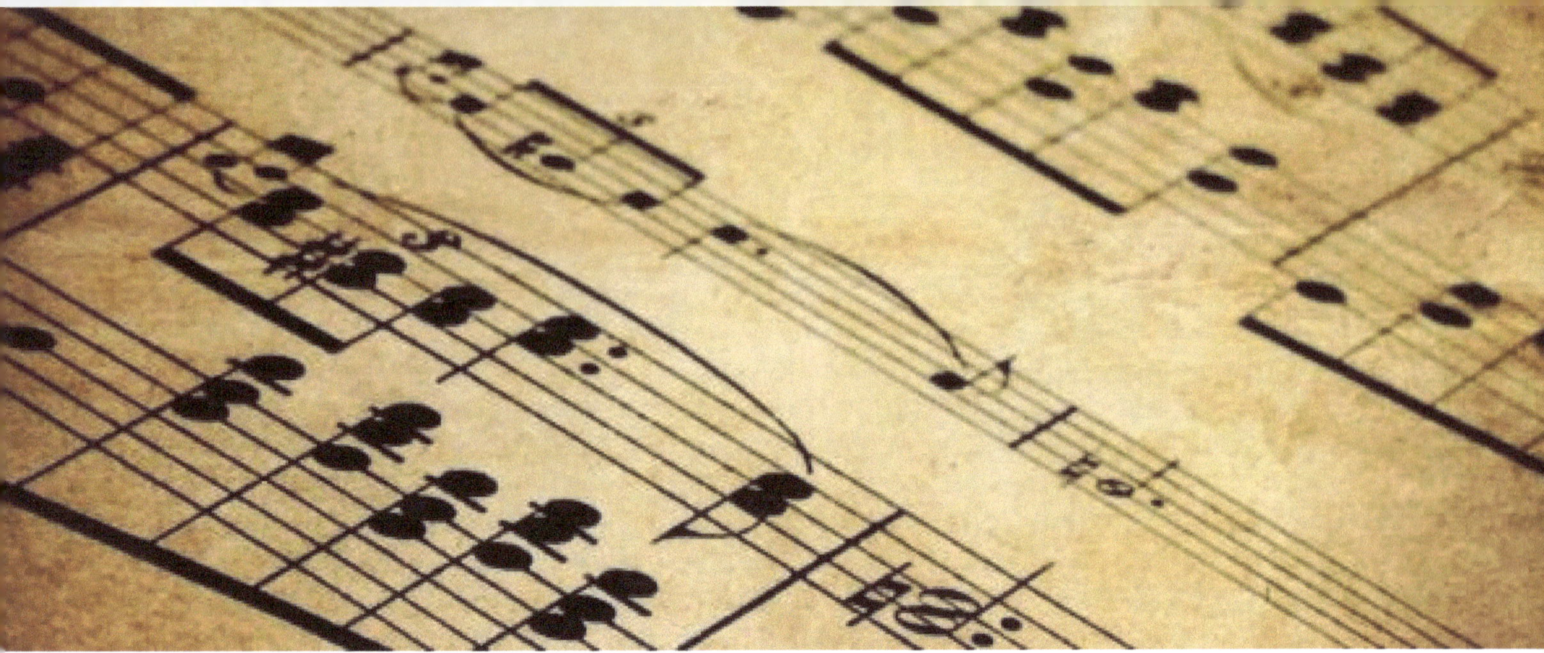

Music Matters
By Ted Stachulski

I recently attended a Music Matters presentation with ten fellow survivors and a handful of caregivers. Genni, a Music Therapy Intern at the Portsmouth Music Arts Center, was invited to run the group.

She placed several percussion instruments on a table, and members got to choose which one they wanted to play during the 45-minute session. I saw tambourines, bells, and different types of drums and rattles I'd never seen before. All were uniquely shaped, and many were very decorative. I realized that out of the vast assortment of instruments, there would be at least one to match everyone's disability. I needed to find the one that fit mine.

There were instruments you could play with one hand or two hands, some you could hold in your hand and shake, or those which could be placed in your lap and hit with your hand or a stick. Each of them made different types of sounds such as loud, soft, high pitch, low pitch, rattling, pounding and ringing. There were so many choices it sent my damaged frontal lobe into overload!

I took a deep breath and thought about my issues with loud noises that startled and overloaded me. I also thought about how my left hand becomes easily fatigued and painful in a

> "I realized that out of the vast assortment of instruments, there would be at least one to match everyone's disability."

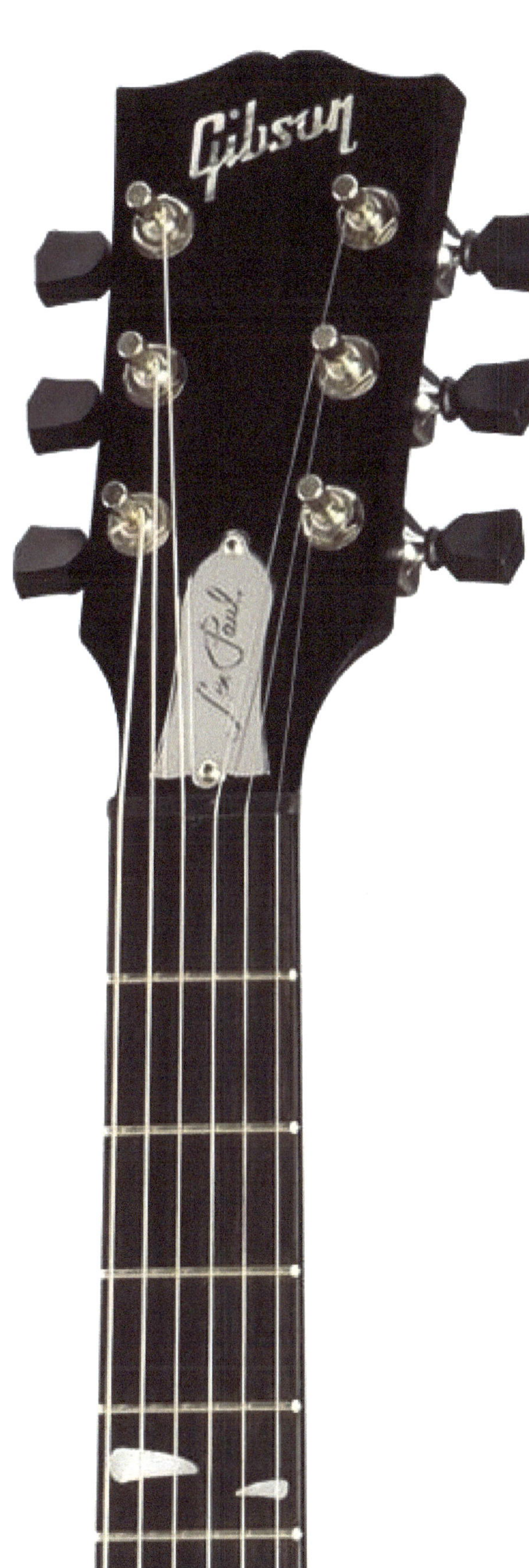

short period (which often leads to me dropping things.) I took another look around the table and carefully chose a small, egg-shaped shaker that made a pleasant sound. I picked it because it fit perfectly in the palm of my hand and I could use either hand to play it. I felt pretty confident that I didn't have to worry about accidentally dropping it or launching it across the room.

As members filtered into the room, they picked up an instrument and sat in a circle. Genni explained to us that music therapy is important in the recovery of brain injury because it lights up parts of the brain, which are involved in movement, planning, attention, learning, and memory. The brain releases chemicals and makes connections on both sides of the brain. In doing so, music helps improve a person's quality of life and promotes healing.

Several members shared how music helped them with memory, sequencing, auditory processing, concentration, mood, anxiety, motivation, positive thinking, meditation, recalling memories, and reducing pain and stress.

Genni warmed us up with some rhythmic exercises where she played a beat on a drum and then we repeated it with our percussion instruments. This gave members a chance to get familiar with their instruments and change to another one if it wasn't the right match for them.

She then picked up a beautiful, midnight blue colored acoustic guitar and began playing and singing the song, *Listen to the Music*, by the Doobie Brothers. Members drummed along to the beat and sang out loud. The song filled my mind with happy thoughts of how I persevered to improve the quality of my life and became involved with the wonderful people at the Krempels Center.

Not all of the beats were played on time, and the notes weren't sung in perfect pitch, but as I listened intensely, I noticed Genni had the voice of an angel. She was being accompanied by a group of fallen angels with brain injuries and some caregivers who were playing instruments and singing their hearts out as if they were on the stage of Carnegie Hall. It was like heaven on earth!

Genni then handed members a piece of paper with the lyrics to the song, Changes, by David Bowie. She proceeded to play it, and people sang aloud.

Wow! I was blown away by the lyrics, and they made me instantly think about my long and weary brain injury journey. Even though I had changed due to my Traumatic Brain Injury, I struggled for many years to try and live my life as the old me. I kept looking inward expecting me to be the same person I was before the accident, but what I always saw was a stranger. I didn't like that stranger then and sometimes I still don't like him now!

Even worse, I tried with all of my might to be the old me, which invariably failed. Some people who knew me before my accident thought I was faking my injury. Whether I wanted to or not, and regardless of what anyone else thought, I had become a different man, and the changes were permanent. Every minute of every day, I struggle to accept that.

> **"Some people who knew me before my accident thought I was faking my injury."**

My happy mood slowly dissipated and became replaced with sadness. Tears from a million old emotions, thoughts and failures from living a lifetime with brain injuries began to fill my eyes. Memories of days gone by filled my mind — from being a child racking up concussions playing tackle football, serving in the military, working and doing my best to raise a family. How I falsely learned from an older generation of men what it took to be a man, how to deal with and resolve problems with violence, and never letting anyone know how I feel.

I realized it was all a bunch of bull! I should've been taught:

• Value and protect my brain as if it was the universe because injuring it could result in permanent damage or recovery that could take a long time.

• Long-term quality of life is more important than playing games which can damage the brain through concussions and a multitude of sub-concussive hits.

• It's okay to talk about your feelings and resolve conflicts without violence.

The group continued to sing.

"Ch-ch-ch-ch-changes (Turn and face the strange)
Ch-ch-changes Don't tell them to grow up and out of it
Ch-ch-ch-ch-changes (Turn and face the strange)
Ch-ch-changes Where's your shame
You've left us up to our necks in it
Time may change me
But you can't trace time."

I thought about a previous discussion on shame and guilt I had attended a while back in the same classroom. All my life I've been buried up to my neck in shame and guilt because of my brain injuries when I shouldn't have been. The people who were supposed to look out for me and my safety should be ashamed of what they did to me and others when we were children!

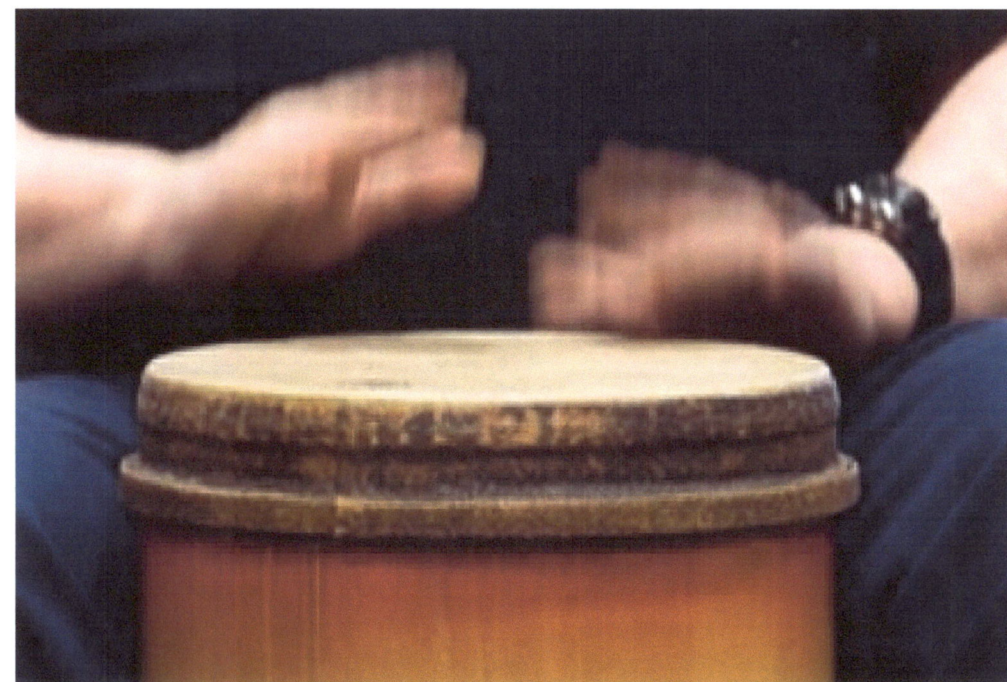

Traces of every hit, emotion, memory, feeling and abuse (verbal and physical) had been permanently embedded and crisscrossed through my mind, body, and soul. Each one of them had an impact on my family members, friends, co-workers, and others.

Traces felt and seen within me by an assortment of therapists I had been to over the course of my life. Their horrified gasps, which from time to time uncontrollably leaped out of their mouths, didn't go unnoticed by me.

From Traumatic Brain Injury to muscle memory to physical and emotional trauma, we worked together to learn how the tangled mess inside of me happened and then decided on which strategies I could use to live a better quality of life as I moved forward in recovery.

When I snapped out of the thoughts that had consumed me, Genni had redirected the group to another activity with the song, *Count on Me*, by Bruno Mars.

I looked around the room and saw happy faces singing, swaying bodies using their instruments to make percussive sounds, and friendship.My tears began to dry up and my mood greatly improved. I then put Music Therapy into my toolbox of strategies I could use to improve the quality of my life as I moved forward in recovery.

No matter what life has thrown at me thus far, I'm glad the changes in my life (good and bad) have led me to the Krempels Center, where I have many friends, interns, and staff I can count on to get me through the next stages of my life. It is a place where members can share their stories to teach other members, interns, and staff about the complexities of their brain injuries and which therapies work best for them.

Meet Ted Stachulski

Ted Stachulski is a former multi-sport athlete, Marine Corps Veteran, Traumatic Brain Injury Survivor, creator of the Veterans Traumatic Brain Injury Survivor Guide, Veterans Outreach Specialist and an advocate for brain injury survivors, their family members and caregivers. In 2007, he received the State of Vermont Governor's Certificate of Appreciation / Traumatic Brain injury Survivor of the Year award for his outstanding commitment, perseverance and advocacy within the brain injury community on a local and national level.

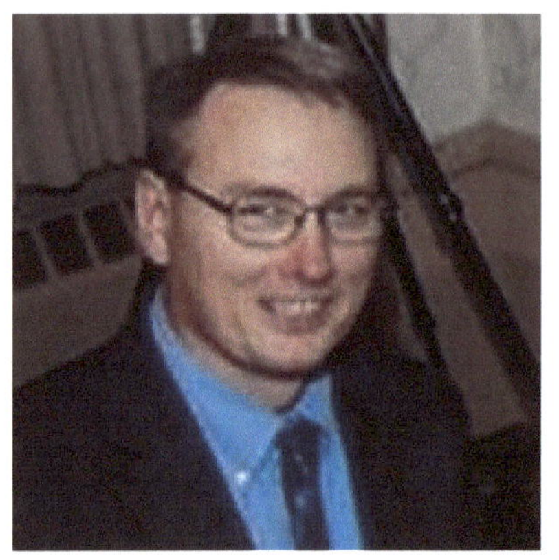

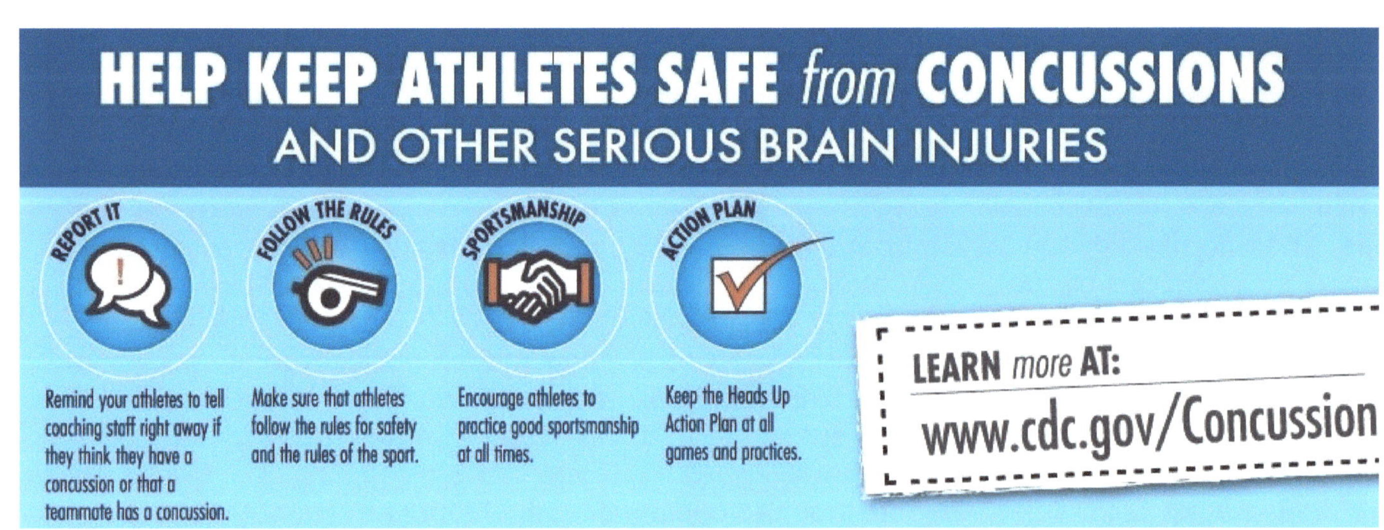

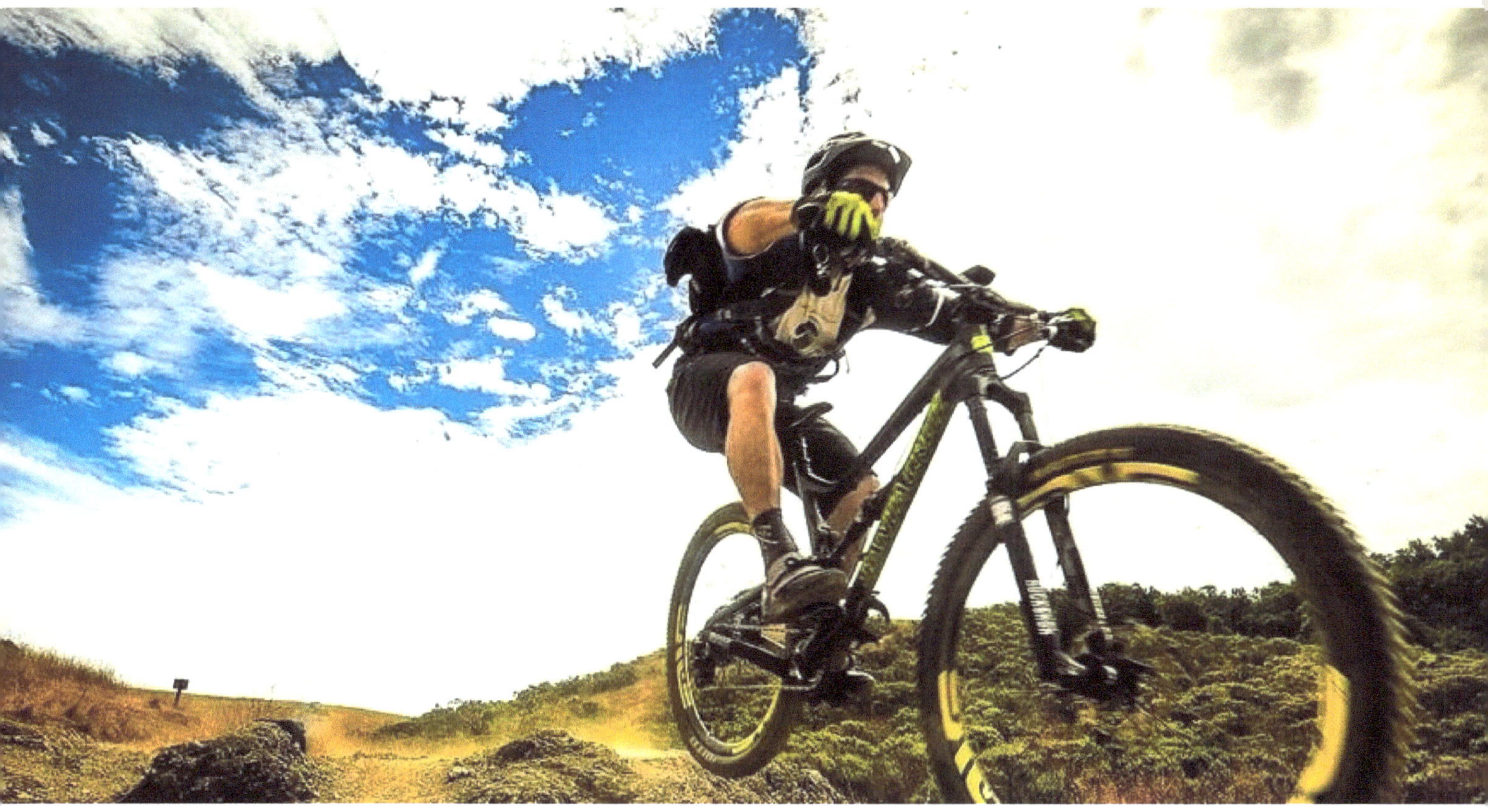

Life after Brain Injury
By Darron Eastwell

The last three years have gone by so fast for me. On May 23, 2015, I joined a club that no one wants to join. It has millions of members worldwide from all different countries and walks of life. The club I'm talking about is the Brain Injury Survivor Club, which carries a life membership. I joined due to a mountain bike accident in which I have zero memory of, nor the subsequent months of being in hospital.

The injuries that I sustained were horrific, including a fractured skull, fractured neck, and fractured T7 in my spine, with the worst being my brain injury. Diagnosed with a severe Diffuse Axonal Injury, the injuries were so severe that I was placed in a medically induced coma for ten-days in the Intensive Care Unit. The treating doctors advised my family that there was a high chance that I might not wake up from the coma and that if I did, there was a high chance that I would be in a vegetative state.

I eventually came out of the coma to the surprise and joy of my family and the treating doctors. I could walk, talk, and function - not the same as before the accident, but I could pretty much function.

> "The injuries that I sustained were horrific, including a fractured skull, fractured neck, and fractured T7 in my spine, with the worst being my brain injury."

The next two months were spent in three different hospitals completing Brain Injury Rehabilitation. Treatment included occupational therapy, speech therapy, balance group, and physical therapy. I was discharged after two months of aggressive treatment. Once I was out of hospital, I had to continue my rehabilitation therapies as an outpatient. For another twelve months, I was constantly challenged, but I would keep on saying to myself "you have to keep going." My family was my biggest motivator and support.

I was sick of hospitals and the routine of rehab, and I just wanted to be back to my old self, doing the things that I loved. Until one day I just said to myself "Darron stop looking backwards at what you could do before your TBI, you have to look forward and look at what you can do today, be thankful you are alive, you can walk, talk and laugh and you are surrounded by family that loves you." This was the moment for me that I felt the change of getting better. It was the time I accepted this new Darron, the TBI Survivor. Mindset is everything.

I had tired of the traditional rehab therapies that I had been doing since I was a patient, and now as an outpatient, so I spoke with my wife Bianca about a plan to try new rehab and become even more motivated in getting better. We both agreed that the therapists had done as much as they could do, and I had put in as much energy and effort as I could. I needed a break and a change in focus. We decided that I should leave rehab and commence our own rehab ideas.

I joined a local gym that was close to my home so I could go on a regular basis. My theory was that having a healthy body equals a healthy mind.

Early on, Bianca went with me to the gym to keep an eye on me and make sure I was ok. After about six months I decided I could walk there and actually made it to the gym!

The next stage that I wanted to reach was to ride my bike to the gym. After about twelve months of gym work and increasing my fitness levels, the big day came to get back on my bike and attempt to ride to the gym.

The feeling of cycling to the gym was great. It was another step forward in my recovery and helped me gain some independence back. I was still not medically cleared to drive a vehicle, so my new vehicle was the trusty mountain bike the one that I crashed on.

Over the past three years, I have slowly been able to increase the time and effort I spend in

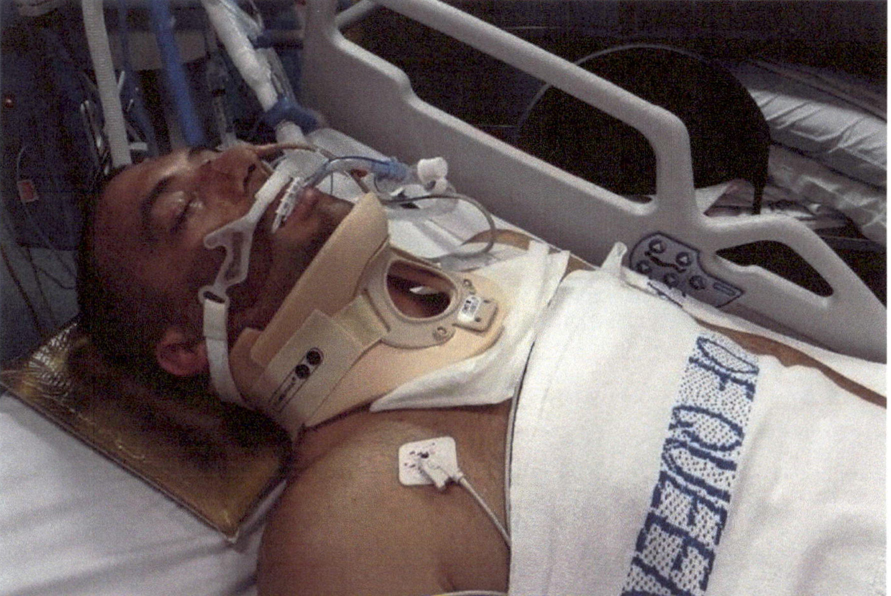

the gym: early on, I spent thirty minutes and now I am able complete a solid two-hour session. This includes riding to and from the gym as well as a solid workout routine that could include rowing, running, strength and conditioning weight training.

Walking our family dog on a regular basis was another new therapy for me. Our family dog is such a beautiful soul. She is a black and white border collie named Remi. Not only did she provide company while walking, she also helped put a smile on my face. As they say, dog is man's best friend. I now know that family pets assist with healing.

Bianca, my wife, is very knowledgeable with natural remedies. She wisely suggested that I start doing basic yoga, meditation, and Yoga Nidra practice at night to assist with my sleeping issues. I practiced Yoga during the day when I was home alone in a quiet place. At first, I found it to be very difficult understanding what to do but, sure enough, it became easier over time.

Meditation is a life skill that anyone can learn. All you need is to make the time and find a quiet place. Over the journey, I have started meditation while down at the local beach, laying on the floor at home in a dark room, or when I go to bed at night. The best kind of relaxation for me was the Yoga Nidra / sleep meditation practice that Bianca suggested we do each night when we go to bed.

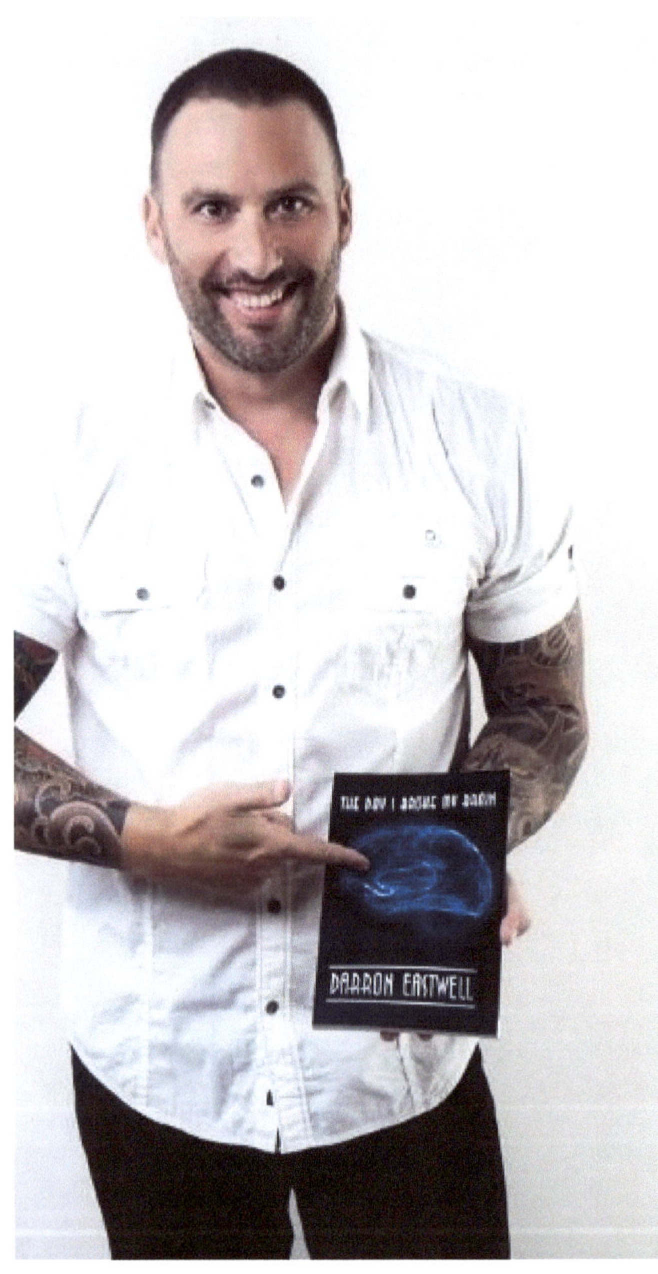

It is a 20-30 minute relaxation where you are listening to a person talking calmly about relaxing every part of your body. I highly recommend this practice for everyone, even those without a TBI. Be patient with yourself and give it a go.

I also cleaned up my diet and made more of an effort to eat healthy "brain foods" more often, as well as eliminating alcohol from my diet. I had my first drink of alcohol since my accident at our family Christmas lunch this year. It was only a celebratory drink and I can comfortably say I am still not a drinker. I am better without it.

I am using essential oils to help ease some of my TBI issues, especially my daily brain fog and constant headaches. I have been able to eliminate all prescribed medication and only use natural supplements, along with the essential oils.

Without a doubt, one of the best things that I have been able to accomplish since my TBI changed my world was writing my first book and becoming a published author. My first book is titled *The Day I Broke My Brain*.

Writing and reading was something that I did not do on a regular basis prior to my TBI. In fact, the last time I did it on a regular basis was when I was at High School for English some twenty-five years ago.

One of the suggested therapies was to start writing a daily journal about what I did or was supposed to do. This would assist me with my memory and fine motor skills like writing, reading, spelling, and remembering what words to use to explain my emotions, thoughts and express myself. Over twelve months of writing, this daily journal evolved into my first book.

I contacted David Grant from Hope Magazine and asked if he could read my first draft manuscript. By June of 2017, the book was complete. Not only have I been able to write my first book, but I have also established my own website, www.darroneastwell.com.au, and a blog. This helps improve my writing.

I have also started my public speaking journey and was invited to speak at a few local events where I live. I speak about my journey and recovery in hopes to inspire others. Another form of therapy that I have tried during my recovery is music therapy. I have been taking guitar lessons now for the past twelve months. It was something that I always wanted to do, but did not have the time for. Thanks to my TBI, I can now play the guitar. I can assure you, I am no rock star, but I can play a few songs and riffs – I just love it. In fact, I completed my first public gig where I played in front of about a hundred people.

My favorite therapy, however, is ink therapy. I was always interested in tattoos but never seemed to have the time to get them. In April of 2015, I finally made the decision and the commitment to get some serious ink completed. I started to search for a tattooist in my local area who specialized in my favorite style of tattoo - Japanese style. The majority of tattoos that I like come from Japanese mythology, but my mountain bike accident and recovery stalled the new ink while I recovered.

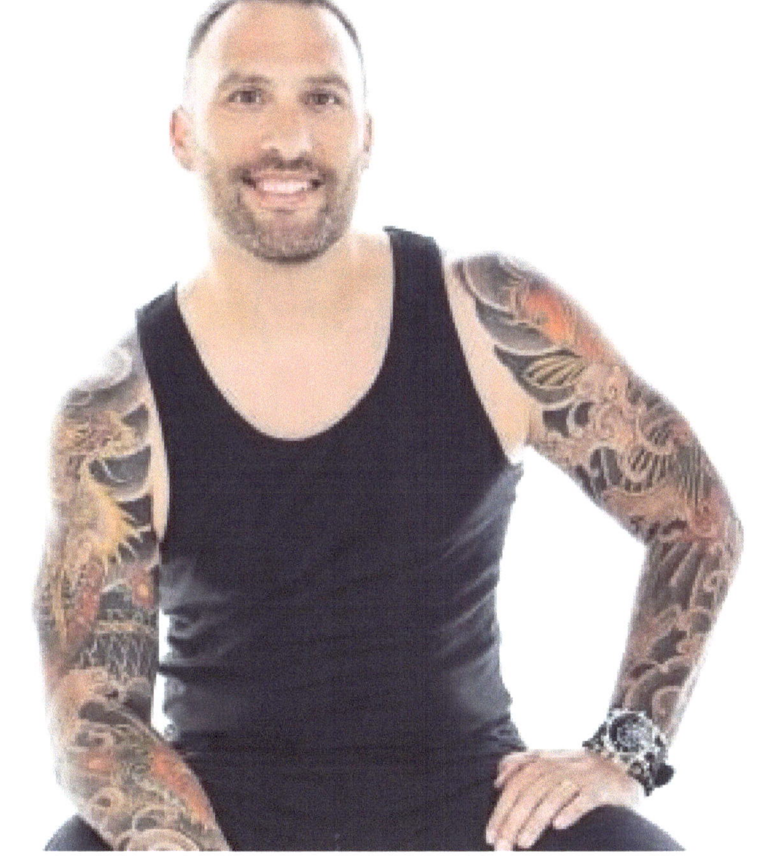

I must admit, I was quite anxious, as it had been about twenty years since my first tattoo. I could not remember the pain and feelings from that time. Given my TBI condition, I was not sure how I would be able to cope with the concentration, fatigue, noise or pain. Much to my surprise, I have to describe the tattoo process as being the best kind of experience I had undertaken since my accident.

The adrenaline took over and I was amped up with excitement. There was no pain from the needle in the tattoo gun, rather a constant blunt massage sensation. The noise didn't bother me either. My concentration was good, although having great conversations helped, along with listening to music that I loved, and laughing throughout the tattoo session. I was having the best time of my post TBI life.

I described getting tattooed as my favorite therapy. I had plenty of sessions to go to and I look forward to plenty more in the future. Now both of my arms and my back are fully tattooed in the Japanese style.

My near death experience and life-changing traumatic brain injury have given my family and me so much negativity, stress and anger over the past three years. However, I can honestly say that the many positives easily exceed the negatives.

I am able to appreciate my life so much more. I enjoy the simple little things that I did not have time for before my TBI and I can laugh so much more these days. I have been able to achieve so much because of my TBI. I get to spend much more time with my loving family than I did before my TBI.

Back before my injury, I was a corporate banker. I was working ridiculous hours, constantly setting goals for promotions and earning more money to climb the corporate banking ladder. None of this matters any longer. I live in the very moment, which is a very beautiful and calming thing. I love my life – I am one of the lucky ones. I have learned that mindset is everything.

Meet Darron Eastwell

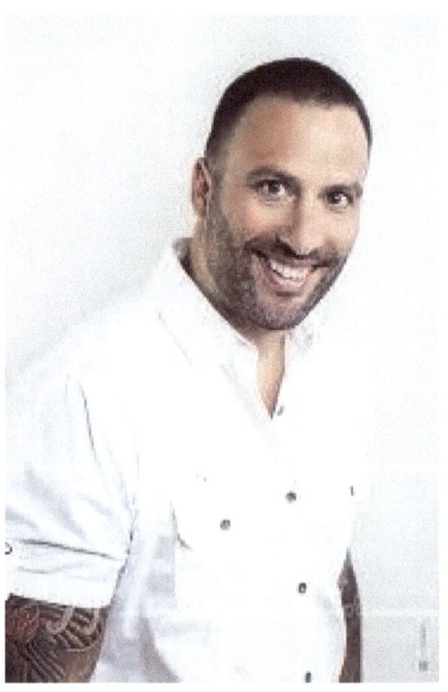

Darron Eastwell is a brain injury survivor from Australia. Darron sustained his injury while mountain biking, an injury he was not expected to recover from. Darron has surpassed all medical expectations of his recovery and now advocates on behalf of those with brain injury.

He is a published author, public speaker, and tireless advocate for those who need a voice. His first book, The Day I Broke My Brain, is available on Amazon. You can learn more about Darron, and read his blog at www.darroneastwell.com.au

> ## "Great works are performed not by strength but by perseverance."
>
> *~Samuel Johnson*

News & Views 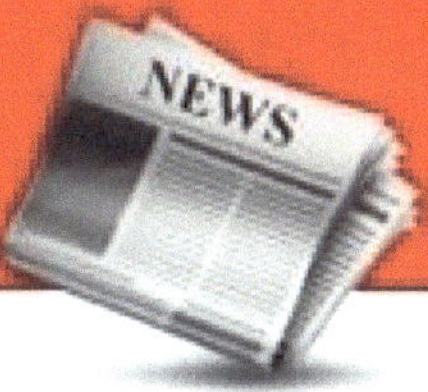

You have just read some inspiring stories about survivors who have found a way, against seemingly insurmountable odds, to reshape their lives, and to begin anew. Entire families are affected by brain injury and are often shattered when brain injury becomes part of daily life. This is not an easy road. Just ask anyone who has had a life after brain injury of any kind.

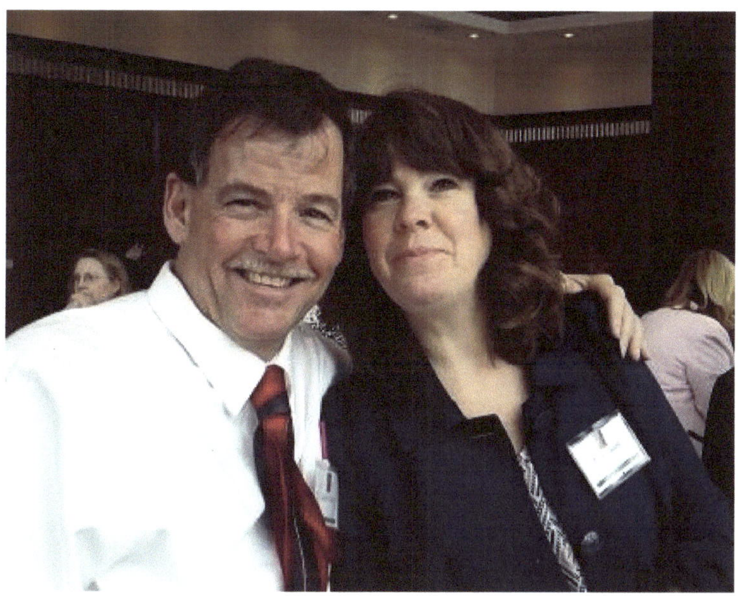

We are always trying to find new ways to share resources, information, and help with others who share our fate as a survivor family. In our own case, we have found that peer-to-peer support has been an invaluable part of our ongoing recovery. We have not walked alone in our journey since the first year post-injury.

If you have found something helpful in your own recovery, we would love to hear from you. Whether it has been a compensatory strategy, a treatment protocol, or something you never envisioned as being helpful to you, we would love to hear about it.

Send us an email to info@tbihopeandinspiration.com to tell us about it.

To this month's contributors, a heartfelt thank you. If you have been thinking of sending your story for publication consideration, now is the time!

May you find peace in your journey,

~ David & Sarah Grant